THE ORIGINAL W

Edward Davy "

THE
ORIGINAL WRITINGS OF

Edward Bach

Compiled from the Archives of the
Dr Edward Bach Healing Trust, Mount Vernon, Sotwell.

By Judy Howard and John Ramsell
Curators and Trustees.

SAFFRON WALDEN
THE C.W. DANIEL COMPANY LIMITED

First published in Great Britain in 1990
by The C.W. Daniel Company Limited
1 Church Path, Saffron Walden
Essex CB10 1JP, England.

ISBN 0 85207 230 9

Designed by Peter Dolton.
Designed and produced in association with
Book Production Consultants, Cambridge, England.
Typeset by Anglia Photoset, Colchester, England.
Printed in England by
St. Edmundsbury Press, Bury St. Edmunds, England.

CONTENTS

The photograph on page ix was taken by Mechthild Scheffer.

FOREWORD

It is our great pleasure to present this book, a compilation of Dr. Bach's original writings, in order to share with you some of his most inspirational teachings.

Edward Bach devoted his entire life to healing, and after nearly twenty exhausting years of research, he eventually discovered a new method of healing using trees, plants and flowers, each specifically selected for their ability to treat the emotional outlook and personality of the sufferer. The Bach Flower Remedies are now used by millions of people all over the world, their successful growth having been established and firmly anchored by their efficacy alone.

It was always Dr. Bach's policy to publish his findings without delay, and to replace these publications with a new account as each milestone was reached. He wanted this system of healing to be as simple to understand as possible so that self-treatment with the remedies would be within reach of people of all walks of life. His booklet "The Twelve Healers & Other Remedies" is the definitive record of his life's work, and is therefore the most authoritative text as it contains all the information necessary to select the remedies for oneself. This booklet and "Heal Thyself", Dr. Bach's philosophy, are available individually and will be familiar to most of you, so to avoid unnecessary repetition, they have not been re-printed in this volume. Neither have we included the earlier publications in the "Twelve Healers" series, namely "The Twelve Healers and the Four Helpers" and "The Twelve Healers and the Seven Helpers", nor Chapter 12 of Free Thyself as this too made reference to his first recordings. Dr Bach referred to these as the "scaffolding" of his final and completed work, and because some of the descriptive states were re-written during the natural development of his discovery, and may therefore become misleading for future readers, it was Dr. Bach's express wish that these old descriptions should not be re-published (see page 139). We do, however, present to you many of Dr. Bach's most stimulating philosophical compositions, letters and lecture notes, and a collection of many other papers which reflect his personality, thoughts and intentions. Together they provide a most wonderful insight and appreciation of a man whose humility and compassion are a blessing to us all.

We feel sure you will enjoy this collection of writings, re-printed from the originals kept in our archives at Mount Vernon, and we hope it will bring to you as much pleasure as it has given us.

John Ramsell and Judy Howard,
Curators and Trustees of:
The Dr. Edward Bach Healing Trust and Centre,
Mount Vernon, Sotwell, Wallingford, Oxon.
OX10 0PZ, England.

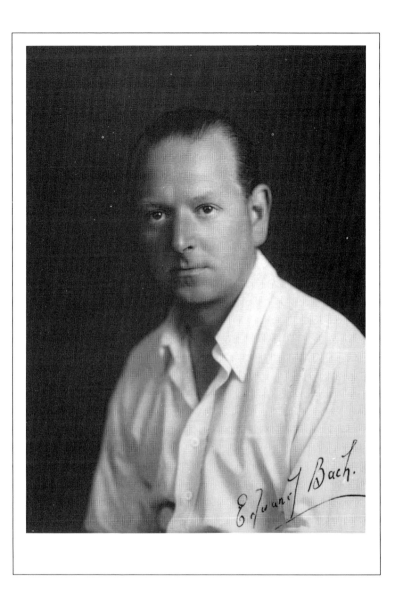

Introduction

We have introduced and explained each chapter of this book separately to guide you through the various stages of Dr. Bach's career, but as a general introduction, we have selected a resumé of his life and work, written by Nora Weeks who was his closest helper, companion and chosen successor, and who therefore knew his work intimately. The doctor's full life story is told in her biograpy *The Medical Discoveries of Edward Bach Physician.*

EDWARD BACH, PHYSICIAN, BACTERIOLOGIST –
DISCOVERER of the HEALING ESSENCE in FLOWERS.

by Nora Weeks

Born, in 1886, not poor but hesitated to put his father to the expense of a medical training.

Eventually his father learned of his son's strong urge towards healing and readily provided the means for him to enter Birmingham University in 1906. From there he went to London to finish his training at University College, where he qualified in 1912.

Only his intense enthusiasm for for the art of healing kept him in London, for city life was a misery to his nature. His gratitude to his father prevented him from asking for money and he spent more on books than would allow to feed himself adequately.

Though he applied himself to his books he spent more time on the close study of every patient and proved to himself many interesting facts about diseases. One conclusion he arrived at was that the same treatment did not cure the same disease. He decided that the personality of the patient was of more importance than the bodily condition, although, of course, this could not be ignored. Years of recording of his studies of individuals, together with his extensive knowledge of an original research into bacteriology, led him 20 years later to discover a new system of medicine.

Like many another genius he placed all his learning in the background and followed his own intuition. This reliance on his inner conviction quickly developed to become a constant attitude which he held and followed implicitly.

Ill health in 1913 caused him to give up the post of Casualty House Surgeon. When he recovered he took consulting rooms in Harley Street. Then he became interested in the immunity school and took a post as assistant bacteriologist. During this work he produced new vaccines which were successful in many cases of arthritis.

During the 1914 war he worked himself to death and collapsed. Skilful surgery brought him to life, but he was told he had only three months to live. In spite of, or rather, in view of this dire news he returned in a very weak state to take charge of the laboratories. After some months forgetting his disabilities in the pressure of work he grew stronger. Friends who saw him later were astonished to see him alive. He himself concluded that it was the awareness of a purpose in his life that brought him back to health.

His successful findings in intestinal toxaemia were published in the

Proceedings of the Royal Society of Medicine for the year 1920. But he was still not satisfied. He therefore fitted up a lab. of his own. Later he obtained the post of Pathologist and Bacteriologist at the London Homoeopathic Hospital. There he read Hahnemann's great work and felt that he was now on the scent of what he was looking for. However, he felt that there was something beyond Homoeopathy and that he would find it in the plants and trees.

He did nothing by halves. In 1930 he gave up his £5,000 a year occupation and devoted all his time to seeking for herbal remedies. Intuitively he knew that these remedies had to be non-poisonous. In fact from now he discarded his scientific knowledge and the methods of Science and trusted entirely to his sensitive intuitional faculties. For six years he proceeded on these lines, finding a few remedies each Summer and healing sick people in the Winter. He used only the flowers of the plants and trees having found a way of potentising the flowers by the rays of the Sun.

His equally revolutionary discovery, worked out in great detail by close observing of individuals, was that it was not the disease that needed treating, but the moods and characteristics of the personality of the patient.

Having found 38 remedies and cured hundreds of people; and having written two booklets stating his scheme simply and clearly, he died peacefully in 1936.

His work is being carried on by a group of his friends, whose address is:

The Dr. Edward Bach Healing Centre,
Mount Vernon,
SOTWELL,
Wallingford,
Berks.

CHAPTER I

THE EARLY YEARS

Edward Bach has become most well-known and revered for his discovery of the Flower Remedies, but during the course of his medical career, he accomplished a great deal of important and highly respected work in relation to intestinal toxaemia which eventually formed the basis of the Homoeopathic Bowel Nosodes which he developed with John Paterson M.B.

> *"On the staff of the University College Hospital.*
> *Lecturer to London University.*
> *Chief bacteriologist to the London Homoeopathic Hospital.*
> *Own consulting practice in Harley Street. Own research laboratories in Park Crescent, London, where he had a permanent staff of four doctors.*
> *Very large practice, over 700 doctors from all parts of the world sought his advice, many came to be trained by him in his laboratories.*
> *He made many discoveries, both in general medicine and homoeopathy, all of which have been published in medical journals and books, and are being used by doctors all over the world."*
>
> *Nora Weeks.*

This early work represented a major milestone in Dr. Bach's medical discoveries because it became the platform from which his ideas of healing with the flowers of the countryside evolved.

Dr. Bach wrote many papers and books, some in association with his colleagues, Dr. Charles E. Wheeler, Dr. T. M. Dishington and Dr. Paterson, but only those most relevant to his future discoveries have been chosen to be included herein because it is the Flower Remedies upon which we wish to concentrate. That was the result of his life's work and therefore superseded in importance all that he had previously achieved.

The following papers do, however, illustrate how his work matured. The third paper entitled "The Discovery of Psora" will be of particular interest as it takes us to the very brink of his search for the healing flowers.

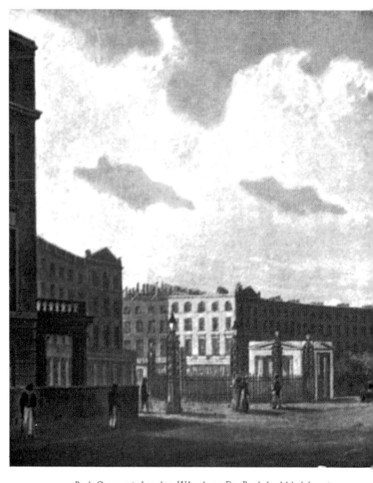

Park Crescent, London W1 where Dr. Bach had his laboratory.

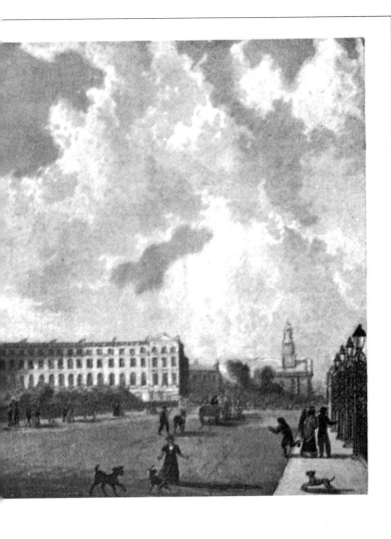

The Problem of Chronic Disease.

By Edward Bach, M.B., B.S., D.P.H.

From the earliest records of medical history we find evidence that what we know to-day as intestinal toxæmia was consciously or unconsciously recognized, as evidenced by the drugs and remedies used by the earliest physicians, many of which were laxative and liver stimulating and hence intestinal cleansing in their effect. Throughout the ages of medical science similar efforts by different methods have been attempted, and even today much of modern treatment by diet, drugs, and even surgery is based on similar conceptions.

The alimentary canal must of necessity be of the utmost importance. Its superficial area is greater than that of the skin surface of our bodies; moreover, it has the power of absorbing from that in which it is bathed – a property not possessed by our external surface in any similar degree; you may sit in a bath of potassium cyanide with no ill-effects, a very small amount of which would be fatal in the stomach; you may wash in water loaded with typhoid or diphtheria or other bacilli without harm, but if a microscopical amount enters the mouth the result may be serious or fatal.

The content of the tract is the fluid in which we live; from which we obtain our fluid and our food; it is to us similar to the water in which the unicellular amœbæ moves. It is essential that it should be pure and contain the necessaries of life, and free from any substances which if absorbed may be harmful to the body and against which there is no protective mechanism.

It is surely one of the marvels of Nature that she has been able to cope with such diversity of intestinal content as that with which different races have tested her powers of adaptation. Consider the varying diets of different countries; think of the vastly varied composition of the intestinal content as a result; and yet the races, generally speaking, survive. As yet the penalty is not death – merely disease; not extinction – merely degeneration.

In all probability the human race was originally intended to live on raw material, the fruits and foods of the tropics, and the human alimentary canal was evolved to deal with such a diet; yet offshoots of that race have migrated to temperate climes and many nations live almost entirely on food which has been cooked, completely altering the intestinal content – and yet the race survives; but humanity does not escape entirely. It may live, but if suffers; it suffers from a hundred and one diseases, from a lowered standard of health and strength and a loss of physical vitality.

It is against all probability that human nature will for some time if ever retrace its steps and return to a primitive condition, and even if that ultimately is the result it does not concern us; we are interested in those countless millions of this, our age, and the age of the near future, who will demand to live as we do to-day and yet cry aloud for health and relief from suffering. We have to meet present needs, not stand idly waiting for an ideal future.

When a race lives on unnatural food, the intestinal content changes chemically, physically and bacteriologically. All these factors matter, but in people such as those with which we are dealing the bacteriological change matters most.

The chemical and physical characters can be brought somewhat within range of normal by a diet not too far removed from that of civilization by the addition of fruit, salad, &c., and by such means the extreme variance from the normal in both the chemical and physical condition can be remedied even within the limits of diets which are not incompatible with the modern possibilities of private home and public restaurants. I mean that it is possible to lunch and dine daily at many restaurants and select such food as will keep the intestine reasonably clean without being considered mentally deranged or even very exceptional. But although this may be accomplished it does not of necessity follow that it is in itself sufficient to cure disease.

In a few cases it may be so, but where there has been an infection of long standing, or where the infection is deeply seated, the bacterial element will resist for at any rate a long time the improvement in the intestinal content, and other methods have to be devised to hasten its removal; hence the greater importance of the bacterial infection as opposed to the abnormal chemical and physical state, owing to the greater difficulty in correction.

Has it ever occurred to you what difference there is between the content of the large intestine of an individual living on raw food and one living on cooked food?

In the latter instance such as is met with in civilized people the content is foul in odour, dark in colour, alkaline in reaction; containing many products of putrefaction such as indol, and the bacterial content is composed of *Bacillus coli*, streptococci and spore-bearing organisms. Contrast this with the healthy individual who lives on raw material.

The large intestinal content is of no odour, light in colour, acid in reaction; free from putrefactive products, and the bacterial content consists of the lactic acid bacilli together with some *Bacillus coli*.

To any conversant with this contrast it is in itself grounds for serious thought.

In many cases cure can be accomplished without alteration of even an unnatural diet, where no amount of dieting would give marked benefit, though I do not deny that the combination would be better and more lasting.

The essential point about a suitable diet is that whilst supplying the needs of the body it should tend to keep the reaction of the large intestine slightly acid – instead of alkaline, as is much more usual in western civilization. The acidity depends on the growth of the lactic acid bacillus, and this organism, again, needs the presence of starch to ensure its multiplication. Ordinary forms of starch are converted to sugar long before the colon is reached, but uncooked oatmeal, or better still, crushed nuts, are convenient means of supplying a starch that remains largely unconverted to sugar in the upper part of the bowel.

I do not feel that it is yet proven that the class of bacteria which is the subject of this paper are the cause of disease. I am not certain. They may be the result, but I do maintain that this group of organisms of which I am about to speak are persistent in patients; that they are associated with chronic disease, and that by the use of preparations made from these bacteria themselves we have a most powerful weapon in the fight against chronic disease of all types.

I turn now to the consideration of these organisms, indicators of potential, if not of present, disease whenever they are found, and found they can be in the vast majority of our fellow citizens. It may be asked why, if they are so deadly, is disease not always demonstrable? The answer is that their immediate virulence is small, and bodies that start with a reasonable measure of health can face their toxins for years without apparent inconvenience. But as life advances with all its various stresses the strain of keeping back these organisms, or possibly the conditions which give rise to them, begins to tell, and presently there is a breach in the defences and obvious illness declares itself. It is because a breakdown can normally be deferred until middle age, when the next generation is launched, that resistance to these organisms is not a very active power, for it remains often true that Nature, if careful of the type, is careless of the single life. In a similar way the long latent period of tuberculosis led to the belief held for many years that it was not infective.

The germs of which I speak are bacilli – Gram-negative, of the great coli typhoid group; the important point being that they are incapable of fermenting lactose – a point which distinguishes them from the *Bacillus coli* itself.

They are not pathogenic in the ordinary sense, as are the typhoid or dysentery or paratyphoid bacilli, and have in the past been mostly regarded as of no importance. They are not identical with but closely allied to these organisms, and belong to their class.

Their number is probably enormous, possibly infinite. It is possible to investigate a hundred without obtaining two identical strains.

We can, however, put them into groups, though even this is relatively a crude classification, as it must be understood that each group contains a host of varieties, differing from one another in some minute detail.

For the purpose of this work these non-lactose fermenting bacilli have been attached to one of six groups, namely:–

Dysentery.
Gaertner.
Faecalis alkaligenes.
Morgan.
Proteus.
Coli mutabile.

They are grouped according to their powers of fermenting certain sugars, and only a few sugars have been used so as to keep the number of groups small. If an autogenous vaccine is used the exact definition of the organism is of no importance for treatment, and the polyvalent throws a very wide net and contains many representatives of each class.

These, then, are the bacilli which for the most part are considered harmless, but which are really the indication and, if properly used, a means of cure of chronic disease.

The clinical evidence of the power to cure is too well established to admit of doubt, and will be referred to presently, but the laboratory is accumulating evidence of a non-clinical nature which demonstrates the connection between these organisms and disease.

By daily examinations of the fæces of a patient it is possible, by recording the percentage of organisms present in the form of a chart, to show the relation between the condition of the patient and the percentage found.

By percentage I mean the ratio between the abnormal non-lactose-fermenting organisms and the number of *Bacillus coli* present. Generally speaking, it is considered normal for coli alone to be present, but these abnormal bacilli may be found in anything from 1 to 100 per cent. of the total colonies obtained.

From the alteration in percentage during treatment it can be ascertained to a certain degree how well a patient is likely to respond.

As a general rule the organisms found remain true to type for any given case. That is to say, Gaertner does not seem to change to a Morgan or a proteus.

If a patient's fæces are plated daily and the percentage of abnormal bacilli charter, it will be found that these are not uniformly present, but that they occur in cycles. Perhaps for a period the specimens are free, and then the organisms appear, rapidly rise in numbers, remain at the highest point for some time, and then diminish until they disappear.

The intervals of freedom from them, the periods of the positive phase of their presence, the highest percentage of them reached, vary in different cases, but the clinical condition of the patient bears a certain relationship to the curve of organisms present in the specimens.

This relationship is not yet sufficiently worked out to lay down definite laws, as more than one type of curve exists; but I can assure you there is a definite relation between clinical conditions and bacterial percentage, and as an example of this the most brilliant result after vaccine treatment occurs when there is a short negative phase followed by a higher and more prolonged positive phase than that which is the patient's usual routine. Generally speaking, those cases where there is little or no alteration from their usual type of course do not do so well.

Much work has still to be done on these lines and it will lead to a profitable result.

It is extraordinary how rapidly the bacterial content may alter. Perhaps after weeks of negative plating, within thirty-six hours the specimens may contain as high as 100 per cent. of these abnormal bacilli.

What happens to produce this result we do not yet know; whether these organisms kill off the normal coli, whether the coli become altered to the abnormal type, whether it is a changed condition of the intestinal content or of the patient himself that causes this change gives room for much research, and when that problem is solved we shall have made a great advance towards the knowledge of the cause of disease.

But whatever may be the explanation, it is already established that the percentage of these bacilli in the specimens bears a direct relation towards the condition of the patient in his varying phases from a clinical point of view.

Another curious feature is the stability of a particular type of bacillus in a given subject, to which I have already alluded. Over several years, no matter how often examinations be made and whatever the condition or disease of the patient, the particular type remains true. Moreover, it is rare to find more than one type in the same case, although this may happen in a small percentage.

There are certain symptoms which occur more frequently with one type than with another, and it is not improbable, when further observations are made, that it will be found there is a close relationship between certain disease symptoms and definite types of these organisms.

Whether these organisms be the cause or result, they are associated with chronic disease, and an enormous amount of benefit can be obtained by the use of vaccine made from them. This has certainly been proven conclusively during the last twelve years.

I have previously referred to the fact that the clinical evidence of the value of this method of treatment is sufficient to leave no room for doubt. That statement must be justified.

Hundreds and thousands of patients have been treated on these lines, by a considerable number of practitioners; by both hypodermic and potentized preparations. Eighty per cent. of those patients have shown improvement (to place it at a moderate figure), some only a little benefit, the majority very definite relief, a good many brilliant results and about 10 per cent. practically miracles.

It is not without years of experience and experiments, not without the observation of thousands of cases, that I place this proposition before you; not without the co-operation and observation and experience of practitioners throughout the British Isles, who will support this evidence.

Patients may be treated with vaccines of these organisms given by hypodermic injection, as has been done now for a considerable number of years. This does not concern us to-day, but I may refer you to our book, "Chronic Disease," for details.

The point I wish to stress is that as good, and I and others believe better, results are obtained by potentized preparations of killed organisms.

These have been in use for about seven years, and extensively for the last two years, by homœopaths and allopaths alike, and there are allopaths who have discarded the syringe for their use.

These potencies may be of two varieties, autogenous and polyvalent. I want to make this point quite clear.

An autogenous preparation means that the bacillus of a particular patient is potentized and used for that patient.

A polyvalent implies collecting organisms from some hundreds of patients, mixing together and potentizing the whole. It is this preparation which has been submitted to you on previous occasions, as a nosode worthy of your consideration.

The autogenous is of use only for the subject from whom it was prepared, or possibly any patient having an identical infection. The polyvalent, on the other hand, is prepared with the object of covering as many cases as possible.

Of the relative merits of the two more experience is yet necessary before we can draw definite conclusions, but that is not of the utmost importance at this point, because even if the autogenous should be shown to give a higher percentage of good results, the polyvalent variety is so successful as to be a nosode worthy of consideration as an additional nosode for the homœopathic materia medica, and the results obtained by any who try this will be sufficiently good (I can say with confidence) that if it ever fails they would probably be stimulated at least to try the autogenous, and thus comparative experience will accumulate in a suficient degree to be able to draw conclusions.

Work is being done on this subject at the present time, but it will be some time before a definite statement can be made. It is hoped that by various tests it will be possible to ascertain whether the polyvalent, autogenous, or even a mixture of two or three strains, will be the perfect form of administration for any particular patient.

It is necessary that I should delay you for a moment, that this paper may be complete, to give you the exact technical details of preparation so that any competent bacteriologist can prepare these potencies.

Fæces are plated on MacConkey's ribipel agar, incubated sixteen hours. When this is done organisms grow as red or white colonies. If they ferment lactose with the production of acid, that acid reacts on the neutral red in the medium to give a red colony; if they be non-lactose fermenters no acid is formed, no action on the neutral red and the colonies grow white. Hence the only interest is in those colonies which after incubation are white in colour.

Cultures made from white colonies, rejecting the coloured, on agar slopes, incubated fifteen hours and sugar reactions determined to group the organisms.

One culture washed up in 2 c.c. distilled water.

Sealed and killed at 60° C. for thirty minutes.

Triturated with milk sugar, the whole in 9 or the whole in 99 grm. of milk sugar.

This makes 1st decimal or 1st centesimal potency, according to the amount of milk sugar used. Further potencies are made by trituration up to the 6th c or the 12th x, and thereafter with the usual fluid mediums.

Special care is necessary in sterilizing all apparatus used to free them of a previous potency. Dry heat of at least 140° C. for 15 minutes is probably more effective than steam or moist heat.

The polyvalent nosode is obtained by collecting cultures from several hundreds of cases; by adding them as they are obtained to a sterile bottle, and when a sufficient number has been reached 1 c.c. of the whole well mixed and shaken is potentized as above.

As far as my knowledge goes there is nothing in this nosode contrary to the laws of Hahnemann, and as a single remedy I believe it is more comprehensive than any other single one known.

It is a link between the allopathic and homœopathic schools; discovered by a member of the allopathic vanguard, it is found to be in line with homœopathic principles.

I submit this nosode to you as a remedy worth including in your pharmacopœia; useful especially as a basic remedy in cases which fail to respond to ordinary drugs, or where no remedy is especially indicated, though its use need not be restricted to these cases.

Much work has yet to be done; experiments are now being conducted to attempt to find whether these organisms are the cause or effect of the patient's condition.

The nosode I submit to you is being tried in both America and Germany, and in this country it is being used by a considerably larger number of allopaths than homœopaths. Some of the former, who for years have been getting good results with the hypodermic variety of the vaccine, have completely discarded the syringe in favour of the potency.

I believe that the proper use of this nosode is to regard it as a basic remedy, and I have no doubt that the most brilliant results will be obtained when it is followed by homœopathic treatment, matching the symptoms with the appropriate remedy.

The nosode is capable of removing a greater or less amount of a really profound basic trouble. It, so to speak, purifies the patients and tends to clean them up until they clearly express one simillimum, and renders them much more responsive to their remedy. Hence, brilliant though the results are which have been obtained by allopaths, in your hands they should be even better.

I appeal to you to give the nosode a trial – to use it on cases who have failed under other treatment and in those cases where a remedy is not clearly indicated. I can speak with confidence that you have only to give it a trial to find it very valuable.

I am not laying too much stress on the autogenous because I know that the polyvalent as a nosode will appeal to you more readily. In the case of giving vaccines hypodermically it is almost essential to have an autogenous to get the best results; here 95 per cent. of the patients do much better on their own vaccine and only about 5 per cent. respond more definitely to the polyvalent; but in the case of this potentized variety it is yet too early to make any such claim, and such is the success of the polyvalent that I am inclined to think in some cases it is better than, and in a large majority of cases equally as good, as the autogenous, though there probably will be always certain cases that will only respond to a personal nosode prepared from their own organisms.

The nosode, the remedy prepared from the material of disease, antedated bacteriology and the vaccine; but the relation of the latter to the former is obvious. To your school, pioneers in the clinical use of disease to cure disease, I offer a remedy which is, I believe, potent against the deepest of all diseases, that chronic toxæmia which the genius of Hahnemann divined and named. If I believe that I can make its nature clearer than was possible for him, I take no jot from his glory – rather I believe I am confirming and extending his work, and so paying him the only homage he would desire.

Reprinted from "Medical World," January 24th, 1930.

An Effective Method of Preparing Vaccines for Oral Administration

BY

EDWARD BACH, M.B., B.S.(LOND.).

During the last ten years a new method of preparing vaccines for oral administration has been thoroughly explored, extensively used and beyond all doubt proved to be of great therapeutic value in cases of chronic disease. A large number of practitioners in the British Isles, America, Germany, France and other countries can testify to the value of this method to such an extent as to leave no doubt that an important therapeutic agent has been added to the materia medica of our science.

There are such definite advantages in the oral method of administration of vaccines that any advancement in this direction must naturally be welcomed by practitioners and public alike. Firstly, one of the great drawbacks of hypodermic injections is the necessity of adding antiseptic, a substance which all of us would wish to avoid introducing into the tissues. Secondly, very many patients have a distinct antagonism to vaccines in the usual form and are thus debarred from the benefits of this form of therapy; they have, however frequently no objection whatever, when the preparation is given orally. Thirdly, the pain and swelling of local reaction is entirely avoided, and in most cases general reaction is markedly less, a matter of considerable importance to those of low vitality and to the aged. Fourthly the danger of sepsis or of accidental infection, though of course this is extremely rare, is completely removed. Fifthly, these preparations are much less costly, and their use may be extended to those who cannot afford the expense of an autogenous hypodermic vaccine.

Up to the present time, although a certain amount of work has been done on acute disease with every promising results, attention has been mainly concentrated on all forms of chronic disease in which intestinal toxaemia has been wholly or in part the cause, and several hundreds of cases have been investigated. The relation to chronic disease of the non-lactose-fermenting organisms found in the intestinal content has now been so definitely established and accepted so universally by bacteriologists that no further comment on this point is necessary in this paper. The acceptance is of a two-fold nature:— firstly, that these organisms play an enormous part in predisposing the patient to chronic disease of almost every form; secondly, that vaccines of these bacilli are valuable therapeutic agents and that great benefit has been obtained by their use. Suffice it to say that a vast amount of disease, heretofore considered hopeless, has been brought within the reach of cure.

The number of varieties of these non-lactose-fermenting bacilli is great – certainly amounting to thousands, if they are examined in minute detail according to the sugar reactions etc., but from the point of view of therapeutic administration of oral vaccines it is sufficient at the present time, at any rate, to divide them into seven main groups, classified according to their reactions on four sugars, as in the following table:—

	GLUCOSE	LACTOSE	SACCHAROSE	DULCITE
Faecalis alkaligenes	Alkaline	—	—	—
Dysentery type	Acid	—	—	—
Morgan type	Acid & gas	—	—	—
Gaertner type	Acid & gas	—	—	Acid & gas
Proteus type	Acid & gas	—	Acid & gas	—
Coli mutabile	Acid & gas	Late Acid & gas	—	—
No. 7 type	Acid & gas	—	Acid & gas	Acid & gas

For the purposes of treatment there are two requirements: (1) a bacteriological investigation to ascertain if the patient has an infection with any of the above types of organism, and (2) an autogenous vaccine, or the polyvalent vaccine of the particular group to which the infecting organism belongs.

To determine if any intestinal infection is present, the faeces of the patient are plated in the usual way, using McConkey's neutral-red-bile-salt-peptone-lactose agar. If white colonies are present, these are picked off and cultures made, which are tested on the four sugars, as shown in the table above, to ascertain into which of the seven groups they fall. It must be borne in mind that these abnormal organisms are not persistently present and that positive and negative phases occur, exactly as they do in the case of typhoid carriers, so it is often necessary to make daily examinations until a positive result is obtained. As a rule three or four examinations are sufficient, but occasionally it is necessary to continue for a few weeks; a longer time than three weeks is uncommon.

The method of preparation is as follows: An 18-hour incubated agar slope of the organism is washed up in 2 c.c. of distilled water, and the emulsion killed in the ordinary way in the water bath at 60°C., except that thirty minutes is sufficient, instead of the usual hour. 1 c.c. of this emulsion is added to 99 grammes of milk sugar in a mortar and the mixture is vigorously ground with a pestle for twenty minutes. The resulting powder is the first strength of the vaccine. 1 gramme of this powder is then added to 99 grammes of milk sugar and similarly ground for twenty minutes: this gives the second strength. 1 gramme of this is then added to 99 grammes of milk sugar and similarly ground to give the third strength, then 1 gramme is added to 99 c.c. of distilled water and vigorously shaken in a bottle; this gives the fourth strength. The process is continued by adding 1 c.c. of this mixture to 99 c.c. distilled water and again well shaking; and so on for any number of times, with repeated dilution and succussion.* The strengths which are most frequently used are the twelfth and the thirtieth.

For the preparation of a polyvalent vaccine it is necessary to obtain a large number of cultures of the particular group, keeping these until at least a hundred have accumulated, thoroughly mixing them, and then taking 1 c.c. of the mixture and treating it as above. Thus it is possible to have a powerful vaccine of each of the seven groups pure to strain.

---

* One-half or one-quarter of all these amounts may be taken, if found more convenient, provided the proportion is maintained.

Method of Dosage.

It has been found that with old people and debilitated subjects, or with cases where a definite reaction is undesirable, it is better to commence with a dose of the twelfth, but with the more vigorous it is quite safe to begin with the thirtieth stren'gth. The dose consists of 3 or 4 drops taken from the stock bottle and added to 1 oz. water; this should be given in two halves at four hours' interval, preferably before food. It is then essential to await the result, allowing at least three weeks to elapse before deciding that no benefit has been obtained. If any improvement occurs, no matter how slight, no further dose should be given under any conditions whatever as long as the least progress is being made, even though this may mean waiting weeks or months only repeating when the condition becomes definitely stationary, or there is a tendency to relapse.

Illustrative Cases.

Case 1. Miss N. G. aet. 35. Epilepsy. Attacks started at six years of age, averaging one a week. Mother epileptic; father alcoholic. Bacteriological examination of faeces gave 20 per cent. of an abnormal bacillus of the Morgan type.

October 28, 1927. First dose of twelfth strength. Improvement followed. No sign of any trouble for a period of almost six weeks, when a very mild attack occurred,

December 7th, 1927. Dose repeated.

February, 6th, 1928. Very mild attack. Third dose given.

The case is still under observation. In all, twelve doses have been required in nearly two years, the last being given in May, 1929. There have been five definite attacks during that period the last one being on November 21, 1928. During 1929, the most serious symptoms have been slight giddiness and depression on four occasions.

Case 2. Mr. J. L. aet. 44. Chronic colitis of five years standing; frequent loose stools with much mucus exacerbations with attacks of diarrhoea every three or four weeks. General debility with marked depression and frequent headaches. Bacteriological examination of faeces gave 90 per cent. of an abnormal bacillus of the proteus type.

June 22, 1928. First dose of thirtieth strength given. Rapid and marked improvement, with disappearance of all symptoms by the end of July. Patient remained well until March 1929, when there was a slight return of symptoms. The dose was repeated, again with rapid improvement, which has been maintained.

Case 3. Mr. C. J. aet. 50. Nervous breakdown due to overwork and business strain; marked depression and inability to concentrate, steadily increasing during one year; nervous dyspepsia, pain and flatulence following food. Bacteriological examination of faeces gave 5 per cent. of an abnormal bacillus of the Morgan type.

August 8, 1927. First dose of thirtieth strength. Steady improvement, and by the middle of August patient able to resume light duties. Progress continued, and by the middle of September patient considered himself unusually well.

October 1, 1927. No further progress, so second dose given. Still further improvement, and condition better than for some years.

Owing to slight relapses four more doses were given during the next eight months, the last being on June 22, 1928. Since then there has been no necessity for any treatment.

Case 4. Mrs. B. aet. 62. Severe headaches, debility, and other symptoms of chronic renal disease. Blood pressure 232.

Examination of urine showed albumen and casts present.

Bacteriological examination of faeces gave 10 per cent. of an abnormal bacillus of the faecalis alkaligenes type.

January 3, 1928. First dose of twelfth strength. General improvement. headaches less frequent and severe. Blood pressure fell to 209. Amount of albumen diminished.

February 4, 1928. Second dose given, as condition appeared stationary.

A further three doses were given in 1928, and two in 1929. The headaches have almost entirely disappeared since April, 1928, and the general health has been good, the blood pressure keeping about 200 and the percentage of albumen slight.

Case 5. Mrs. C. aet. 44. Very severe headaches for eight years, one a month, necessitating at least one day in bed.

Bacteriological examination of faeces gave 2 per cent. of an abnormal bacillus of the Morgan type.

January 14, 1928. First dose of thirtieth strength.

The February attack was missed.

March 8, 1928. A mild attack necessitated a second dose.

Since then six further doses have been given, the last one being on April 19, 1929. For the last twelve months the attacks have been very mild and have now practically ceased.

It will readily be seen that the great advantages of this method of administration apply not only to the patient, but also to the physician, because once good stocks of polyvalent vaccine have been prepared, they are practically inexhaustible. Hence the cost is reduced, and the administration is easily carried out by any practitioner. The only necessary preliminary is a bacteriological examination to determine the type of the infecting organism.

So many medical men can now guarantee the efficacy of these preparations that all doubt as to their value has been removed. Hitherto hypodermic vaccines of these abnormal bacilli have very considerably increased our power of cure in cases of chronic disease, and now we have at our disposal an equally effective, but simpler method of treatment, which can be extended to those who have objections or prejudices to the hypodermic method.

Space forbids, in an article of this description, any discussion of the physical properties of these preparations, but the work of modern physicists is tending to show that certain properties are released and that very active substances are present in these dilutions.

This work is being further elaborated by Dr. T. M. Dishington of Glasgow, who has spent several years in patient research on this subject, and it is hoped before long to be able to publish the symptoms peculiar to each particular group of organisms, so that prescribing will be possible on symptomatology alone, without any need of the laboratory.

It will be quite obvious to many of our readers that the method adopted in the preparation of these oral vaccines is identical with that used by the Homeopathic school for the past century in preparing their remedies, and the knowledge that bacteria so treated prove an invaluable therapeutic agent must form a link between the advanced school of Immunity of to-day and that of Homœopathy, which has existed for a hundred years. And although Homœopathy needs no support other than that given by the effective cures obtained through its science, this link must be of great value in demonstrating to members of the allopathic school the confirmation of one of Hahnemann's discoveries by this different point of view which has now been effected in the laboratory.

Reprinted from THE BRITISH HOMOEOPATHIC JOURNAL,

January, 1929.

The Rediscovery of Psora.[1]

By EDWARD BACH, M.B., B.S., M.R.C.S., L.R.C.P., D.P.H.

THE object of this paper is to continue the discussion of the problems presented to you by Dr. Dishington at your last meeting on certain nosodes prepared from abnormal organisms in the intestinal canal, which have been brought before your notice on different occasions during the past eight years. I want to describe to you how these nosodes have been developed and evolved, and the processes of thought, reasoning and practice which have placed them in the position they now hold.

Three main principles had to be realized before the present effective state of these nosodes could be obtained: (1) The discovery of the group of bacilli which formed their basis; (2) the value of Hahnemann's laws with regard to repetition in the application of the doses; and (3) the fact that the nosodes would be effective in a potentized state.

About 1912 it was recognized that there were to be found in the intestinal content of both apparently healthy as well as diseased people a class of bacilli which had hitherto been considered unimportant, but which were then proved to be associated with chronic disease. These organisms were the various types of non-lactose-fermenting bacilli belonging to the great coli-typhoid group, very closely allied to such organisms as the typhoids, dysenteries and paratyphoids, yet not giving rise to acute disease and, in fact, not associated with any specific morbid conditions. Since there was not this connection, they had in the past been regarded as of no importance, and had been disregarded by bacteriologists and clinicians. About this time, owing to the frequency with which these bacilli were found to be

---

[1] Read to the British Homœopathic Society on November 1, 1928.

present in such a large percentage of cases when no other abnormal or pathogenic organisms could be isolated, it was decided to try the use of these in vaccines to see if any benefit could be obtained in cases of chronic disease, and it was found that in spite of them being non-pathogenic in the ordinary sense of the word, great benefit could be obtained when they were used as a therapeutic agent in this manner. It was shown that by such vaccines a mild exacerbation of all the symptoms in a chronic case could be produced, and that in favourable circumstances a definite improvement followed. Cases of good results were recorded when patients were so treated, but in those days the percentage of these was comparatively small, owing to the fact that the injections were given much too frequently and at stated intervals, such as a week or ten days, with a consequent result of serious over-dosing and interference with the starting of a beneficial reaction. At the present time several bacteriologists and a considerable number of clinicians can testify to the undoubted connection that exists between these organisms and chronic disorders and between them and intestinal toxæmia with its consequent morbid results, so that there no longer remains the least doubt as regards this relationship. Some hundreds of practitioners have proved this point from the clinical results that have been obtained by the use of preparations made from these organisms, and the evidence has now grown so large that there is no longer any room for doubt on this point. A certain amount of laboratory evidence has also been accumulated to prove that there is a relationship between these groups of organisms and disease. If specimens of a patient are plated out day by day for a considerable period, it will be found that these abnormal organisms which are the subject of this paper are not persistently and constantly present, but that there are negative phases when they are entirely absent, and positive ones when they are present in varying proportions. Moreover, the total numbers during the positive phases vary from day to day. If we start plating during a negative phase, after a time they begin to appear in the specimens, at first in small numbers, then steadily rising each day until the maximum is reached, when the percentage again falls until they disappear. Both the maximum percentage and the length of the positive and negative phases may vary very considerably in different subjects, but the interesting point is that the health of the individual, whether in disease or in an apparently normal condition, varies directly with these phases. Most commonly in cases of chronic illness the symptoms are worse towards the end of the negative period and are relieved when there is an output of the abnormal organisms, and generally speaking the greater the output the more benefit the patient receives. In the apparently healthy if there are any times when the individual tends to be below the normal standard and is not up to his usual form, these generally occur at the same period of the cycle. Boyd and Paterson in Glasgow are proving further points of relationship between these states and the condition of the patient.

The result of a vaccine is usually to cause a greater and more prolonged output to the benefit of the patient. If daily charts of the results of the examinations are kept, it is generally possible to know from these the condition of the patients and how they are progressing, and they have very often been a useful guide in selecting the correct time for the repetition of doses. Thus, from a clinical and a laboratory standpoint, there can no longer be any doubt that these groups of organisms bear a distinct relationship to chronic disease.

The next step – the discovery that the doses should be given not at stated intervals, but according to the response of the patient – came as follows: In the laboratories at University College, in treating cases of pneumonia with vaccine, it was found that better results were obtained when doses were given according to how the patient reacted to the injection, and that if after a dose the pulse rate and temperature fell, the results were much more satisfactory if no further treatment was given as long as this improvement continued, repetition only being made when the pulse-rate and temperature tended again to rise. The cures occurred more quickly and with a higher percentage of successful results, and considerably fewer doses of vaccine were required. After this had been definitely realized and proved, it logically followed to try the same method with all types of acute febrile cases, and the same beneficial results were found to occur. When this had been definitely established, it occurred to the same workers that this law which appeared to apply to all acute diseases might possibly be the same for cases of a chronic type. So it was tried, and the results again were more than had been anticipated.

In chronic cases a minimum interval of three weeks was allowed to elapse before a dose was repeated, because it was found that in some instances benefit did not begin much before that time, and if at the end of three weeks improvement had started no further dose was given until every trace of improvement had ceased, and that either the condition had become stationary or there was a tendency to relapse. On these lines it was found that the period of emelioration varied in cases from two or three weeks to intervals as long, in rare examples, as twelve months, and that by refusing to repeat during the time of improvement enormously better results were obtained and a higher percentage of good results occurred, while of course a much smaller amount of vaccine in each case had to be given. Such was the success that this method has been persevered with up to the present time.

At this stage, therefore, we had arrived at two conclusions: (1) That this particular group of non-pathogenic non-lactose-fermenting bacilli of the intestine were undoubtedly associated with chronic disease, and (2) that vaccines made from them were very valuable curative agents, if given according to the laws of Hahnemann and studying the response of the patient, and not, as had hitherto been done, at regular intervals.

It was at this stage that, coming to your hospital as your bacteriologist, one was introduced to the science of homœopathy. On reading Hahnemann's "Organon" for the first time one instantly realized the fact that the work of the modern immunity school was merely the rediscovery, by a different method, of facts that had been realized by him a century before, and in conjunction with some of your physicians homœopathic principles were at once applied to these various groups of bacilli and preparations made from them, potentizing them in the same way as you do your remedies. It required only a very short time to prove that nosodes so prepared were of very great therapeutic value, and the further research of the last eight years, in which many hundreds of cases were treated, has more than justified the earlier hopes. To-day, not only in England, but to an even greater extent in Germany and America, and also to a lesser extent in France, Holland and Switzerland, these nosodes are being used.

Looking at it from the homœopathic point of view, the first important point to be considered is whether these preparations are in accordance with the laws of Hahnemann and whether it is an extension of his work. Many of us feel that this is the case, as the founder of homœopathy in more than one instance uses the morbid product of disease as the basis of a remedy, and one has little doubt that if he had been in a position to isolate these organs they would have been used. Moreover, it is still uncertain whether these organisms are the cause, the result or an attempted cure of disease. We can do little more at the present time than say that there is an association, but its exact nature it is impossible as yet to determine. It is not at all improbable that these bacilli are a variation of the *Bacillus coli*, and the latter, from its universal presence in our modern civilization, not only in men, but in animals, birds, &c., must be considered more or less as a normal inhabitant of the intestine. Experiments tend to indicate that during great basic fundamental changes in the body the intestinal flora may alter, as if attempting to keep in harmony, for it is not impossible that these groups of bacilli are the normal *B. coli* altered to meet certain needs, compelled to do so by the altered state of the host, and that when the bacteria are in this condition they are undoubtedly valuable therapeutic agents when potentized. Science is tending to show that life is harmony – a state of being in tune – and that disease is discord or a condition when a part of the whole is not vibrating in unison.

In a differentiation of these organisms it is interesting to note that the sugar lactose is used. Lactose differs from the rest of the sugars in that it is an animal product, the others being vegetable. Recent research indicates that for a ferment to be able to act upon a substance, the ferment must be able to vibrate in tune with the atomic weight of the substance which has to be fermented. Hence, it means that organisms capable of ferment-ing lactose are able to vibrate in tune with animal tissue, whilst those which are unable to do this are equally unable to be in harmony with substances other than of the vegetable type. If this theory is able to stand the test of time, it will get us a considerable way towards the understanding of things of fundamental nature, and it means that we have here a method of differentiating organisms which are beneficent from those which are adverse to the human subject. It is at such a time as they are adverse that we choose to potentize these products and use them as therapeutic agents in the cure of disease. On all other points, of course, the nosodes are identical with homœopathic remedies, and their preparation is exactly in accordance with the laws of materia medica.

No one who has studied intestinal toxæmia to any extent can possibly fail to see the similarity between this and the basic, fundamental disease described by Hahnemann as psora. I am not going into this in detail to-day, because I understand that Dr. Gordon, of Edinburgh, is going to draw this similarity for you at length at some future date, when he will point out to you the indubitable provings of the nature of intestinal toxæmia which Hahnemann classified under the name of psora.

There is one point of interest which I may mention here in relation to this point, namely, that Hahnemann lays great stress on the impossibility of having more than one disease at the same time. This we find in regard to the work on intestinal flora; it is surprising that only in the very rarest cases does one find more than one abnormal type of organism present in one individual, another point of confirmation of the theory that the two states are identical.

In spite of there only being one type of organism present at a particular period, this type may certainly be changed by means of a vaccine, or nosode, or remedy administration, indicating that the type of organism depends on the condition of the patient, and that it varies its nature in conformity with the soil in which it has to live. Generally speaking, in people who have not been treated by homœopathic methods, the organism remains much more constant to its type over a prolonged period of time.

The next point which has to be emphasized is the extent to which the allopathic school are at the present time adopting homœopathic methods. Quite apart from the work of which I have been speaking this evening concerning these nosodes, which are being used by quite a large number of allopaths in different parts of the world, most of whom have been more or less instructed in the proper principles of repetition, so that no harm is likely to be experienced on that score. There is another school which has quite independently worked out the administration of oral vaccines and is now on a large scale using low potencies of these and giving them by mouth. So far these workers, who are now represented in every country in the world, have not used dilutions above the 4x. During the past few years Besredka and others have done an enormous amount of work proving the efficacy of giving vaccines by mouth, both as prophylaxis against and also as a cure of disease. Large numbers of experiments have shown that animals can be rendered immune against live organisms to which they are very susceptible by a few doses of dead emulsion of the same bacteria given by mouth. Moreover, tests done among troops have very hopeful results as to the power of the same preparations to protect against infection from typhoid, dysentery, &c., in ordinary life, so that at the present time, both for prophylaxis and treatment, the oral vaccine is becoming an established factor and firms are engaged not only in this country, but on a much greater scale on the Continent, in the manufacture of these preparations in large quantities. The suspensions are not potentized in the full sense of the word, but owing to the minuteness of bacteria the total quantity present is very small indeed and probably corresponds to about a 2x or 3x of a homœopathic remedy: hence they are very closely allied to your potencies. This work, which is rapidly growing and extending, comes of course entirely from the allopathic school and has no connection with homœopathy. It has been developed quite independently through scientific laboratories of the old school. Unconsciously, again, Hahnemann's work is being rediscovered, and a vast number of remedies prepared, though only in low potencies. An attempt is being made by the old school to form a complete materia medica, using as their base the various types of organisms, of which of course there are very numerous varieties.

To give you an example, the following is a quotation from the quarterly bulletin of one of our leading firms:–

> "The vaccine-therapist claims a multiple variety of cases in which the use of vaccines by subcutaneous injection is contra-indicated. Acute febrile cases and nervous patients who are hypersensitive may be mentioned as the more important examples.
>
> "It is not generally known in staphylococcal and streptococcal infections oral vaccines, administered by the mouth in the same way as ordinary medicines, are equally

if not more effective than vaccines given by injection. Frequent visits for injections are unnecessary as the patient can easily take the oral vaccines at home at the times ordered by the practitioner. In the treatment of boils and carbuncles some striking successes have been obtained.''

Another aspect which it is necessary for every homœopath to understand is what Habnemann realized well enough – the incompleteness of materia medica and the fact that it could not cover all existing diseases. Moreover, he saw that new illnesses might arise owing to altering circumstances of civilization and that new remedies would have to be sought. Again, his genius comprehended the fact that in Nature might be found an infinite number of remedies to meet all occasions that might arise. The following paragraphs quoted from the ''Organon'' will show you his realization of the necessity for more remedies, and the enormous amount of work that must be done by his followers to improve on his original findings to keep pace with disease in its ever-varying characteristics:–

''Since the number of medicines exactly tested in regard to their positive action is as yet only moderate, it sometimes happens that only a smaller or greater part of the symptoms of a case of disease can be found in the symptom-register of the most suitable medicine. Consequently this incomplete counter-disease force must be employed for a lack of a complete one'' (para. 133.)

''If the drug first chosen actually corresponds to the disease in its entirety, it must cure it. But if, owing to the insufficient number of fully proved drugs and the consequent restriction of our choice, the medicine selected is not exactly homœopathic, then it will arouse new symptoms which will in their turn point the way to the next remedy likely to prove serviceable'' (para. 184).

''Truly only a considerable supply of medicines thus accurately known in their positive modes of action can serve our turn, and enable us to discover a remedy for every one of the innumerable natural cases of disease.

''When thousands of exact and tireless observers, instead of one as hitherto, have laboured at the discovery of these first elements of a rational materia medica, what will it not be possible to effect in the whole extent of the endless kingdom of disease! Then the art of medicine will no longer be mocked at as an art of conjecture lacking all foundation'' (para. 122).

Then again, his realization of the enormous possibilities in the variety of disease is illustrated in the following:–

"Every epidemic or sporadic collective disease is to be regarded and treated as a nameless, individual disorder, which has never occurred before exactly as in this case, in this person and in these circumstances, and can never in this identical form appear in the world again'' (para. 60).

"Every disease epidemic in the world differs from every other, excepting only those few which are caused by a definite unchangeable miasm. Further, even every single case of epidemic and sporadic disease differs from every other, those only excepted that belong to the collective disease noted elsewhere. Therefore the rational physician will judge every case of illness brought under his care according to its individual characteristics. When he has investigated its individual features and noted all its signs and symptoms (for they exist in order to be noted) he will treat it according to its individuality (i.e., according to the particular group of symptoms it displays), with a suitable individual remedy'' (para. 48).

The last point on which one wants to lay stress is that Hahnemann also visualized the inexhaustible supply of remedies if only efforts were taken to obtain them. Quoting from him again:–

"On the other hand, the disease-producing powers usually termed 'drugs' or 'medicines' can be used for purposes of cure, with infinitely greater ease, far more certainty and with a range of choice almost unlimited; we can give to the counter-disease thereby aroused (which is to remove the natural disease that we are called to treat) a regulated strength and duration, because the size and weight of the dose lie at our command; and as every medicine differs from every other and possesses a wide range of action, we have in the great multitude of drugs an unlimited number of artificial diseases ready to hand, which we can oppose with decisive choice to the natural course of the diseases and infirmities of mankind, and so, swiftly and surely, remove and extinguish natural disorders by means of very similar diseases artificially produced.'' (Para. 37.)

There is no doubt that these nosodes are going to play a large part in the future treatment of disease, and if they are essentially homœopathic they ought to be distributed to the world through homœopathic channels for two reasons: (1) That any extensions of Hahnemann's work should be added to that of his which already exists as a natural respect to his genius; (2) a point of far greater importance, these nosodes can only be a perfect success when combined with other homœopathic treatment. It must not be forgotten that these nosodes probably only represent one branch of disease, that included by Hahnemann under the name of psora, and that as a part their action is limited and restricted to a certain phase in the treatment of disease, and cannot be expected under any conditions to cover anything like the whole picture. Therefore, the successful prescriber must also have at his command all other remedies which are at present in the Pharmacopœia or which may in the future be added to it, so that he may be able to deal with the totality of any one or more cases, and whilst the allopathic school is perfectly willing to accept nosodes, or, as they are called, oral vaccines, of bacteria of all forms, it limits the new pharmacopœia to this region of remedies, and will not have the benefit of the hundred years of experience of all the various herbs and natural remedies so completely tested out by your school.

These nosodes may be looked upon as great cleaning powers improving the condition of a patient and in certain cases effecting a complete cure, in others so cleaning up the whole state that the patient, who before gave no response, now receives marked benefit from other remedies. Again, the fundamental factor in using this treatment is the very careful repetition of the doses entirely according to the response of the patient, a law with which all homœopaths are familiar but which it will take a long time for allopaths to appreciate. If these nosodes are launched on the profession through the allopathic world, their chance of success is very small in comparison with what it might be of contracted through your channels, because of these two points, the lack of the complete materia medica and the at present comparatively unknown law of the correct repetition of doses.

Such has been the success of the practical results of these preparations, that already more allopaths have used them than there are homœopaths on the Register in England; some of them have entirely discarded the syringe and the old hypodermic method of injection for the use of the nosode, and one can see a distinct danger ahead if this practice spreads too widely without the control of a ruling body, as it should be used only by men who have had distinct training. The existence of homœopathy in this country depends to an extent on its ability to cure cases where allopathy has failed, and the possession of these preparations enables the allopath who uses them properly to compete to a much more considerable extent than previously, and you can be sure that if this work is taken up by the other school and the proper interval between doses acknowledged, it will be claimed by them as entirely their own discovery. You have to-day in Dr. Paterson, of Glalsgow, your own pathologist working on these nosodes, preparing them and actually doing further research on the subject, so that you are from an internal source proceeding with the work.

In conclusion, I want to remind you of paragraphs which ended a paper I read to you in April, 1920, which are as follows:–

"Meanwhile it should be realized that science in a totally different manner is confirming the principles of homœopathy. To Hahnemann should fall all the honour for having anticipated science by more than a century.

"The attitude to-day of the medical profession in general is one of regard towards homœopathy; but when, as is shortly certain to happen, it is generally recognized and appreciated that all modern research at the hands of allopaths is rapidly proving and drifting in the direction of Hahnemann's laws, then will homœopathy be acknowledged to be the wonderful science that it is.

"Let all the members of your Society see to it that they

are proud to be amongst the pioneers; let them see to it that they do not err one jot from the fundamental laws of their great founder. For science is proving him in detail – the like remedy, the single dose, the danger of hasty repetition.

"It is going to be a struggle between the old homœopathy and the new; see to it that the old receives its due share of credit, that its standard is kept high, and that, true to its teachings, it is not swamped in the flood of science which is merely following in the wake of Hahnemann."

I wish it were possible that we could present to you seven herbs instead of seven groups of bacteria, because there always seems to be some reticence in the minds of many to use anything associated with disease in the treatment of pathological conditions. Possibly this is a narrow-minded outlook, and in this age we are too inclined to want to keep medicine perfectly pure and have swung a little to the opposite extreme, possibly as reaction from the practices of the Middle Ages and the vivisection of to-day. Moreover, it may be that the organisms we are using are beneficent to mankind and not adverse.

We are making every endeavour to replace the bacterial nosode by means of plants and have, in fact, matched some of them almost exactly; for example, ornithogalum in its vibrations is almost identical with the Morgan group, and we have discovered a seaweed which has almost all the properties of the dysentery type, but there is yet one thing lacking, and that one point keeps us checkmated in the effort to avoid using bacterial nosodes. This vital point is polarity. The remedies of the meadow and of nature, when potentized, are of positive polarity, whereas those which have been associated with disease are of the reverse type, and at the present time it seems that it is this reversed polarity which is so essential in the results which are being obtained by bacterial nosodes. Perhaps at some future date a new form of potentizing may be discovered, which will be capable of reversing the polarity of the simple elements and plants, but until that time comes we have no alternative.

The beneficial effect of these nosodes is now accepted internationally, and the daily amount of good which is being accomplished in the fight against disease is on an enormous scale, so that it does not seem that this benefit should be withheld from humanity until such time as we may have found a particular method of combating the psora of Hahnemann by a means which will fit in with the aesthetic mentality of the most fastidious type. Infinitely more important it is that this work should be acknowledged as a continuation of that of Hahnemann and, though not in itself perfect, as leading the way to further discovery. Its growth and development should be watched and directed by the homœopathic school, and not be allowed to fall into abuse in the hands of men who do not understand the fundamental principles on which it is established.

It will interest you to know that three of the plants mentioned on page 32 were Mimulus, Impatiens and Clematis. But in those early days, Dr. Bach prepared the remedies homœopathically, and it was not until he developed the sun and boiling methods of preparation that he was able to overcome the problem of polarity.

The Theory of Groups

The following piece by Nora Weeks, explains the correlation between the Bowel Nosodes and seven type-groups. As he replaced the bacterial nosodes with the flower remedies, these seven type groups formed the seven headings under which specific groups of remedies were placed. Nora Weeks told us how elated Dr. Bach became when he found that he was able to diagnose his nosode treatment more successfully through the personality traits than by clinical tests – for this proved to him that there was undeniably a connection between a person's outlook and temperament and their physical disease.

"In 1928 Edward Bach was searching in every spare moment for the plants and herbs to replace his bacterial nosodes, and one evening he made two vital discoveries about the nature, cause and effect of disease. It happened in this way, he attended a dinner in a large banqueting hall, he went rather unwillingly and was seeking to escape from boredom by watching all the people around him, when it suddenly struck him that the whole of humanity could be classed into groups, or types. Every one of the people in that hall belonged to one of those groups, and he noticed that some resembled one another so closely in their gestures, expressions, tones of voice and other characteristics that they might have belonged to the same family. By the end of the evening he had worked out a number of groups and was comparing them with the seven bacterial groups from which he had already prepared his nosodes, the seven Bach Nosodes, now called the seven Bowel Nosodes. He decided to study seriously the question of these groups.

He wondered how this theory of groups would apply to physical disease and its cure. Would the diseases from which people in the same group suffered be the same? Suddenly he realised that the people in any one group would by no means suffer from the same kind of diseases, but that, whatever disease they contracted, they would react in the same or nearly the same way.

From then onwards he made a practice of observing closely every patient who came to him and began prescribing for them on the basis of the patient's type-group as shown by the moods, mannerisms, habits, reactions to illness and similar indications with his nosodes. The results were so encouraging that now he felt he must be on the right path. The time had come to find the plants and herbs which would heal the patient himself, for then the symptoms, the physical disease, would also be healed."

CHAPTER II

The Middle Years – 1929–1934

"He spent every penny he made on research work, trying by scientific means to find the cure of all disease, especially the so-called 'incurable' diseases. He could not find it this way, so he gave up all his work in London and went into the country to discover a new method of healing and new remedies amongst the simple and divinely provided herbs of the field."

Nora Weeks

Part One

During the next five years, Dr. Bach's travels took him all over England and Wales, from Abersoch to Sussex; the West Country to East Anglia. Each winter he settled in Cromer on the north coast of Norfolk, where he would treat patients in his consulting rooms with his newly discovered remedies. At that time, there were only twelve remedies, which Dr. Bach referred to as "The Twelve Healers", and during this early stage, he thought that all predominant emotional states and personality types corresponded to one of the Twelve Healers. As time progressed, however, he realised that there were certain cases for which he did not have a remedy and so his search continued.

It was during these middle years, between 1929 and 1934, that his early booklets about the remedies were written. His philosophy and descriptions of the twelve remedies were, at first, combined in his initial booklet "Free Thyself" which became the predecessor to both "Heal Thyself" and "The Twelve Healers".

The booklet entitled "Ye Suffer From Yourselves" was an address given to an audience of Homoeopathic doctors. Dr. Bach has often been thought of as being ahead of his time, and his remedies a medicine of the future. In "Ye Suffer from Yourselves" he describes a vision of hospitals and the doctor's role in time to come.

Free Thyself

EDWARD BACH, *Physician,*
M.B., B.S., M.R.C.S., L.R.C.P., D.P.H.

Introduction.

It is impossible to put truth into words. The author of this book has no desire to preach, indeed he very greatly dislikes that method of conveying knowledge. He has tried, in the following pages, to show us clearly and simply as possible the purpose of our lives, the uses of the difficulties that beset us, and the means by which we can regain our health; and, in fact, how each of us may become our own doctor.

Index.

Free Thyself

CHAPTER I.

It is as simple as this, the Story of Life.

A SMALL child has decided to paint the picture of a house in time for her mother's birthday. In her little mind the house is already painted; she knows what it is to be like down to the very smallest detail, there remains only to put it on paper.

The picture is finished in time for the birthday. To the very best of her ability she has put her idea of a house into form. It is a work of art because it is all her very own, every stroke done out of love for her mother, every window, every door painted in with the conviction that it is meant to be there. Even if it looks like a haystack, it is the most perfect house that has ever been painted: it is a success because the little artist has put her whole heart and soul, her whole being into the doing of it.

This is health, this is success and happiness and true service. Serving through love in perfect freedom in our own way.

So we come down into this world, knowing what picture we have to paint, having already mapped out our path through life, and all that remains for us to do is to put it into material form. We pass along full of joy and interest, concentrating all our attention upon the perfecting of that picture, and to the very best of our ability translating our own thoughts and aims into the physical life of whatever environment we have chosen.

Then, if we follow from start to finish our very own ideals, our very own desires with all the strength we possess, there is no failure, our life has been a tremendous success, a healthy and a happy one.

The same little story of the child-painter will illustrate how, if we allow them, the difficulties of life may interfere with this success and happiness and health, and deter us from our purpose.

The child is busily and happily painting when someone comes along and says, ''Why not put a window here, and a door there; and of course the garden path should go this way." The result in the child will be complete loss of interest in the work; she may go on, but is now only putting someone else's ideas on paper: she may become cross, irritated, unhappy, afraid to refuse these suggestions; begin to hate the picture and perhaps tear it up: in fact, according to the type of child so will be the re-action.

The final picture may be a recognisable house, but it is an imperfect one and a failure because it is the interpretation of another's thoughts, not the child's. It is of no use as a birthday present because it may not be done in time, and the mother may have to wait another whole year for her gift.

This is disease, the re-action to interference. This is temporary failure and unhappiness: and this occurs when we allow others to interfere with our purpose in life and implant in our minds doubt, or fear, or indifference.

CHAPTER II.

Health depends on being in harmony with our souls.

IT is of primary importance that the true meaning of health and of disease should be clearly understood.

Health is our heritage, our right. It is the complete and full union between soul, mind and body; and this is no difficult far-away ideal to attain, but one so easy and natural that many of us have overlooked it.

All earthly things are but the interpretation of things spiritual. The smallest most insignificant occurrence has a Divine purpose behind it.

We each have a Divine mission in this world, and our souls use our minds and bodies as instruments to do this work, so that when all three are working in unison the result is perfect health and perfect happiness.

A Divine mission means no sacrifice, no retiring from the world, no rejecting of the joys of beauty and nature; on the contrary, it means a fuller and greater enjoyment of all things: it means doing the house-keeping, farming, painting, acting, or serving our fellow-men in shops or houses. And this work, whatever it may be, if we love it above all else, is the definite command of our soul, the work we have to do in this world, and in which alone we can be our true selves, interpreting in an ordinary materialistic way the message of that true self.

We can judge, therefore, by our health and by our happiness, how well we are interpreting this message.

There are all the spiritual attributes in the perfect man; and we come into this world to manifest these one at a time, to perfect and strengthen them so that no experience, no difficulty can weaken or deflect us fropm the fulfilment of this purpose. We chose the earthly occupation, and the external circumstances that will give us the best opportunities of testing us to the full: we come with the full realisation of our particular work: we come with the unthinkable privilege of knowing that all our battles are won before they are fought, that victory is certain before ever the test arrives, because we know that we are the children of the Creator, and as such are Divine, unconquerable and invincible. With this knowledge life is a joy; hardships and experiences can be looked upon as adventures, for we have but to realise our power, to be true to our Divinity, when these melt away like mist in the sunshine. God did indeed give His children dominion over all things.

Our souls will guide us, if we will only listen, in every circumstance, every difficulty; and the mind and body so directed will pass through life radiating happiness and perfect health, as free from all cares and responsibilities as the small trusting child.

CHAPTER III.

Our souls are perfect, being children of the Creator, and everything they tell us to do is for our good.

HEALTH is, therefore, the true realisation of what we are: we are perfect: we are children of God. There is no striving to gain what we have already attained. We are merely here to manifest in material form the perfection with which we have been endowed from the beginning of all time. Health is listening solely to the commands of our souls; in being trustful as little children; in rejecting intellect (that tree of the knowledge of good and evil) with its reasonings, its 'fors' and 'againsts,' its anticipatory fears: ignoring convention, the trivial ideas and commands of other people, so that we can pass through life untouched, unharmed, free to serve our fellow-men.

We can judge our health by our happiness, and by our happiness we can know that we are obeying the dictates of our souls. It is not necessary to be a monk, a nun, or hide away from the world; the world is for us to enjoy and to serve, and it is only by serving out of love and happiness that we can truly be of use, and do our best work. A thing done from a sense of duty with, perhaps, a feeling of irritation and impatience is of no account at all, it is merely precious time wasted when there might be a brother in real need of our help.

Truth has no need to be analysed, argued about, or wrapped up in many words. It is realised in a flash, it is part of you. It is only about the unessential complicated things of life that we need so much convincing, and that have led to the development of the intellect. The things that count are simple, they are the ones that make you say, ''why, that is true, I seem to have known that always,'' and so is the realisation of the happiness that comes to us when we are in harmony with our spiritual self, and the closer the union the more intense the joy. Think of the radiance one sometimes sees in a bride on her wedding morn; the rapture of a mother with a new-born babe; the ecstasy of an artist completing a masterpiece: such are the moments where there is spiritual union.

Think how wonderful life would be if we live it all in such joy: and so it is possible when we lose ourselves in our life's work.

CHAPTER IV.

If we follow our own instincts, our own wishes, our own thoughts, our own desires, we should never know anything but joy and health.

NEITHER is it a difficult far-away attainment to hear the voice of our own soul; it has all been made so simple for us if we will but acknowledge it. Simplicity is the keynote of all Creation.

Our soul (the still small voice, God's own voice) speaks to us through our intuition, our instincts, through our desires, ideals, our ordinary likes and dislikes; in whichever way it is easiest for us individually to hear. How else can He speak to us? Our true instincts, desires, likes or dislikes are given us so that we can interpret the spiritual commands of our soul by means of our limited physical perceptions, for it is not possible for many of us yet to be in direct communion with our Higher Self. These commands are meant to be followed implicitly, because the soul alone knows what experiences are necessary for that particular personality. Whatever the command may be, trivial or important, the desire for another cup of tea, or a complete change of the whole of one's life's habits, it should be willingly obeyed. The soul knows that satiation is the one real cure for all that we, in this world, consider as sin and wrong, for until the whole being revolts against a certain act, that fault is not eradicated but simply dormant, just as it is much better and quicker to go on sticking one's fingers into the jam-pot until one is so sick that jam has no further attraction.

Our true desires, the wishes of our true selves, are not to be confused with the wishes and desires of other people so often implanted in our minds, or of conscience, which is another word for the same thing. We must pay no heed to the world's interpretation of our actions. Our own soul alone is responsible for our good, our reputation is in His keeping: we can rest assured that there is only one sin, that of not obeying the dictates of our own Divinity. That is the sin against God and our neighbour. These wishes, intuitions, desires are never selfish; they concern ourselves alone and are always right for us, and bring us health in body and mind.

Disease is the result in the physical body of the resistance of the personality to the guidance of the soul. It is when we turn a deaf ear to the 'still small voice,' and forget the Divinity within us; when we try to force our wishes upon others, or allow their suggestions, thoughts, and commands to influence us.

The more we become free from outside influences, from other personalities, the more our soul can use us to do His work.

It is only when we attempt to control and rule someone else that we are selfish. But the world tries to tell us that it is selfishness to follow our own desires. That is because the world wishes to enslave us, for truly it is only when we can realise and be unhampered our real selves that we can be used for the good of mankind. It is the great truth of Shakespeare, "To thine own self be true, and it must follow, as the night the day, thou canst not then be false to any man."

The bee, by its very choice of a particular flower for its honey, is the means used to bring it the pollen necessary for the future life of its young plants.

CHAPTER V.

It is allowing the interference of other people that stops our listening to the dictates of our soul, and that brings disharmony and disease. The moment the thought of another person enters our minds, it deflects us from our true course.

GOD gave us each our birthright, an individuality of our very own: He gave us each our own particular work to do, which only we can do: He gave us each our own particular path to follow with which nothing must interfere. Let us see to it that not only do we allow no interference, but, and even more important, that we in no way whatsoever interfere with any other single human being. In this lies true health, true service, and the fulfilment of our purpose on earth.

Interferences occur in every life, they are part of the Divine Plan; they are necessary so that we can learn to stand up to them: in fact, we can look upon them as really useful opponents, merely there to help us gain in strength, and realise our Divinity and our invincibility. And we can also know that it is only when we allow them to affect us that they gain in importance and tend to check our progress. It rests entirely with us how quickly we progress: whether we allow interference in our Divine mission; whether we accept the manifestation of interference (called disease) and let it limit and injure our bodies; or whether we, as children of God, use these to establish us the more firmly in our purpose.

The more the apparent difficulties in our path the more we may be certain that our mission is worth while. Florence

Nightingale reached her ideal in the face of a nation's opposition: Galileo believed the world was round in spite of the entire world's disbelief, and the ugly duckling became the swan although his whole family scorned him.

We have no right whatever to interfere with the life of any one of God's children. Each of us has our own job, in the doing of which only we have the power and knowledge to bring it to perfection. It is only when we forget this fact, and try and force our work on others, or let them interfere with ours that friction and disharmony occur in our being.

This disharmony, disease, makes itself manifest in the body, for the body merely serves to reflect the workings of the soul; just as the face reflects happiness by smiles, or temper by frowns. And so in bigger things; the body will reflect the true causes of disease (which are such as fear, indecision, doubt, etc.) in the disarrangement of its systems and tissues.

Disease, therefore, is the result of interference: interfering with someone else or allowing ourselves to be interfered with.

CHAPTER VI.

All we have to do is to preserve our personality, to live our own life, to be captain of our own ship, and all will be well.

THERE are great qualities in which all men are gradually perfecting themselves, possibly concentrating upon one or two at a time. They are those which have been manifested in the earthly lives of all the Great Masters who have, from time to time, come into the world to teach us, and help us to see the easy and simple ways of overcoming all our difficulties.

These are such as –

LOVE.	UNDERSTANDING.
SYMPATHY.	TOLERANCE.
PEACE.	WISDOM.
STEADFASTNESS.	FORGIVENESS.
GENTLENESS.	COURAGE.
STRENGTH.	JOY.

And it is by perfecting these qualities in ourselves that each one of us is raising the whole world a step nearer to its final unthinkably glorious goal. We realise then that we are seeking no selfish gain of personal merit, but that every single human being, rich or poor, high or low, is of the same importance in the Divine Plan, and is given the same mighty privilege of being a saviour of the world simply by knowing that he is a perfect child of the Creator.

As there are these qualities, these steps to perfection, so there are hindrances, or interferences which serve to strengthen us in our determination to stand firm.

These are the real causes of disease, and are of such as –

RESTRAINT.	DOUBT.
FEAR.	OVER-ENTHUSIASM.
RESTLESSNESS.	IGNORANCE.
INDECISION.	IMPATIENCE.
INDIFFERENCE.	TERROR.
WEAKNESS.	GRIEF.

These, if we allow them, will reflect themselves in the body causing what we call disease. Not understanding the real causes we have attributed disharmony to external influences, germs, cold, heat, and have given names to the results, arthritis, cancer, asthma, etc.: thinking that disease begins in the physical body.

There are then definite groups of mankind, each group performing its own function, that is, manifesting in the material world the particular lesson he has learnt. Each individual in these groups has a definite personality of his own, a definite work to do, and a definite individual way of doing that work. There are also causes of disharmony, which unless we hold to our definite personality and our work, may re-act upon the body in the form of disease.

Real health is happiness, and a happiness so easy of attainment because it is a happiness in small things; doing the things that we really love to do, being with the people that we truly like. There is no strain, no effort, no striving for the unattainable, health is there for us to accept any time we like. It is to find out and do the work that we are really suited for. So many suppress their real desires and become square pegs in round holes: through the wishes of a parent a son may become a solicitor, a soldier, a business man, when his true desire is to become a carpenter: or through the ambitions of a mother to see her daughter well married, the world may lose another Florence Nightingale. This sense of duty is then a false sense of duty, and a dis-service to the world; it results in unhappiness and, probably, the greater part of a lifetime wasted before the mistake can be rectified.

There was a Master once Who said, "Know ye not that I must be about My Father's business?" meaning that He must obey His Divinity and not His earthly parents.

Let us find the one thing in life that attracts us most and do it: Let that one thing be so part of us that it is as natural as breathing; as natural as it is for the bee to collect honey, and the tree to shed its old leaves in the autumn and bring forth new ones in the spring. If we study nature we find that every creature, bird, tree and flower has its definite part to play, its own definite and peculiar work through which it aids and enriches the entire Universe. The very worm, going about its daily job, helps to drain and purify the earth: the earth provides for the nutriment of all green things; and, in turn, vegetation sustains mankind and every living creature, returning in due course to enrich the soil. Their life is one of beauty and usefulness, their work is so natural to them that it is their life.

And our own work, when we find it, so belongs to us, so fits us, that it is effortless, it is easy, it is a joy: we never tire of it, it is our hobby. It brings out in us our true personality, all the talents and capabilities waiting within each one of us to be manifested: in it we are happy and at home; and it is only when we are happy (which is obeying the commands of our soul) that we can do out best work.

We may have already found our right work, then what fun life is! Some from childhood have the knowledge of what they are meant to do, and keep to it throughout their lives: and some know in childhood, but are deterred by contra-suggestions and circumstances, and the discouragement of others. Yet we can all get back to our ideals, and even though we cannot realise them immediately we can go on seeking to do so, then the very seeking will bring us comfort, for our souls are very patient with us. The right desire, the right motive, no matter what the result, is the thing that counts, the real success.

So if you would rather be a farmer than a lawyer; if you would rather be a barber than a bus-driver, or a cook than a greengrocer, change your occupation, be what you want to be: and then you will be happy and well, then you will work with zest, and then you will be doing finer work as a farmer, a barber, a cook, than you could ever achieve in the occupation that never belonged to you.

And then you will be obeying the dictates of your Spiritual self.

CHAPTER VII.

Once we realise our own Divinity the rest is easy.

IN the beginning God gave man dominion over all things. Man, the child of the Creator, has a deeper reason for his disharmony than the draught from an open window. Our 'fault lies not in our stars, but in ourselves,' and how full of gratitude and hope can we be when we realise that the cure also lies within ourselves! Remove the disharmony, the fear, the terror, or the indecision, and we regain harmony between soul and mind, and the body is once more perfect in all its parts.

Whatever the disease, the result of this disharmony, we may be quite sure that the cure is well within our powers of accomplishment, for our souls never ask of us more than we can very easily do.

Everyone of us is a healer, because every one of us at heart has a love for something, for our fellow-men, for animals, for nature, for beauty in some form, and we every one of us wish to protect and help it to increase. Everyone of us also has sympathy with those in distress, and naturally so, because we have all been in distress ourselves at some time in our lives. So that not only can we heal ourselves, but we have the great privilege of being able to help others to heal themselves, and the only qualifications necessary are love and sympathy.

We, as children of the Creator, have within us all perfection, and we come into this world merely that we may realise our Divinity; so that all tests and all experiences will leave us untouched, for through that Divine Power all things are possible to us.

CHAPTER VIII.

The healing herbs are those which have been given the power to help us to preserve our personality.

JUST as God in His mercy has given us food to eat, so has He placed amongst the herbs of the fields beautiful plants to heal us when we are sick. These are there to extend a helping hand to man in those dark hours of forgetfulness when he loses sight of his Divinity, and allows the cloud of fear or pain to obscure his vision.

Such herbs are –

Chicory	*(Cichorium Intybus)*
Mimulus	*(Mimulus Luteus)*
Agrimony	*(Agrimonia Eupatoria)*
Scleranthus	*(Scleranthus Annuus)*
Clematis	*(Clematis Vitalba)*
Centaury	*(Erythraea Centaurium)*
Gentian	*(Gentiana Amarella)*
Vervain	*(Verbena Officinalis)*
Cerato	*(Ceratostigma Willmottiana)*
Impatiens	*(Impatiens Royalei)*
Rock Rose	*(Helianthemum Vulgare)*
Water Violet	*(Hottonia Palustris)*

Each herb corresponds with one of the qualities, and its purpose is to strengthen that quality so that the personality may rise above the fault that is the particular stumbling block.

CHAPTER IX.

The real nature of disease.

IN true healing the nature and the name of the physical disease is of no consequence whatever. Disease of the body itself is nothing but the result of the disharmony between soul and mind. It is only a symptom of the cause, and as the same cause will manifest itself differently in nearly every individual, seek to remove this cause, and the after results, whatever they may be, will disappear automatically.

We can understand this more clearly by taking as an example the suicide. All suicides do not drown themselves. Some throw themselves from a height, some take poison, but behind it all is despair: help them to overcome their despair and find someone or something to live for, and they are cured permanently: simply taking away the poison will only save them for the time being, they may later make another attempt. Fear also re-acts upon people in quite different ways: some will turn pale, some will flush, some become hysterical and some speechless. Explain the fear to them, show them that they are big enough to overcome and face anything, then nothing can frighten them again. The child will not mind the shadows on the wall if he is given the candle and shown how to make them dance up and down.

We have so long blamed the germ, the weather, the food we eat as the causes of disease; but many of us are immune in an influenza epidemic; many love the exhilaration of a cold wind, and many can eat cheese and drink black coffee late at night with no ill effects. Nothing in nature can hurt us when we are happy and in harmony, on the contrary all nature is there for our use and our enjoyment. It is only when we allow doubt and depression, indecision or fear to creep in that we are sensitive to outside influences.

It is, therefore, the real cause behind the disease, which is of the utmost importance; the mental state of the patient himself. not the condition of his body .

Any disease, however serious, however long-standing, will be cured by restoring to the patient happiness, and desire to carry on with his work in life. Very often it is only some slight alteration in his mode of life, some little fixed idea that is making him intolerant of others, some mistaken sense of responsibility that keeps him in slavery when he might be doing such good work.

There are seven beautiful stages in the healing of disease, these are –

PEACE.	CERTAINTY.
HOPE.	WISDOM.
JOY.	LOVE.
FAITH.	

CHAPTER X.

To gain freedom, give freedom.

THE ultimate goal of all mankind is perfection, and to gain this state man must learn to pass through all experiences unaffected; he must encounter all interferences and temptations without being deflected from his course: then he is free of all life's difficuties, hardships and sufferings: he has stored up in his soul the perfect love, wisdom, courage, tolerance and understanding that is the result of knowing and seeing everything, for the perfect master is he who has been through every branch of his trade.

We can make this journey a short joyful adventure if we realise that freedom from bondage is only gained by giving freedom; we are set free if we set others free, for it is only by example we can teach. When we have given freedom to every human being with whom we are in contact; when we have given freedom to every creature, everything around us, then we are free ourselves: when we see that we do not, even in the minutest detail, attempt to dominate, control, or influence the life of another, we shall find that interference has passed out of our own lives, because it is those that we bind who bind us. There was a certain young man who was so bound to his possessions that he could not accept a Divine gift.

And we can free ourselves from the domination of others so easily, firstly by giving them absolute freedom, and secondly, by very gently, very lovingly, refusing to be dominated by them. Lord Nelson was very wise in placing his blind eye to the telescope on one occasion. No force, no resentment, no hatred, and no unkindness is necessary. Our opponents are our friends, they make the game worth while, and we shall all shake hands at the end of the match.

We must not expect others to do what we want, their ideas are the right ideas for them, and though their pathway may lead in a different direction from ours, the goal at the end of the journey is the same for us all. We do find that it is when we want others to 'fall in with our wishes' that we fall out with them.

We are like cargo-ships bound for the different countries of the world, some for Africa, some for Canada, some for Australia, then returning to the same home port. Why follow another ship to Canada when our destination is Australia? It means such a delay.

Again, we perhaps do not realise what small things may bind us, the very things that we wish to hold are the things that are holding us: it may be a house, a garden, a piece of furniture; even they have their right to freedom. Worldly possessions, after all are transient, they give rise to anxiety and worry because inwardly we know of their inevitable and ultimate loss. They are there to be enjoyed and admired and used to their full capacity, but not to gain so much importance that they become chains to bind us.

If we set everybody and everything around us at liberty, we find that in return we are richer in love and possessions than ever we were before, for the love that gives freedom is the great love that binds the closer.

CHAPTER XI.

Healing.

FROM time immemorial humanity has recognised that our Creator in His love for us has placed herbs in the fields for our healing, just as He has provided the corn and the fruit for our sustenance.

Astrologers, those who have studied the stars, and herbalists, those who have studied the plants, have ever been seeking those remedies which will help us to keep our health and joy.

To find the herb that will help us we must find the object of our life, what we are striving to do, and also understand the difficulties in our path. The difficulties we call faults or failings, but let us not mind these faults and failings, because they are the very proof to us that we are attaining bigger things: our faults should be our encouragements, because they mean that we are aiming high. Let us find for ourselves which of the battles we are particularly fighting, which adversary we are especially trying to overcome, and then take with gratitude and thankfulness that plant which has been sent to help us to victory. We should accept these beautiful herbs of the fields as a sacrament, as our Creator's Divine gift to aid us in our troubles.

In true healing there is no thought whatever of the disease: it is the mental state, the mental difficulty alone, to be considered: it is where we are going wrong in the Divine Plan that matters. This disharmony with our Spiritual Self may produce a hundred different failings in our bodies (for our bodies after all merely reproduce the condition of our minds), but what matters that? If we put our mind right the body will soon be healed. It is as Christ said to us, "Is it easier to say, thy sins be forgiven thee or take up thy bed and walk?"

So again let us clearly understand that our physical illness is of no consequence whatsoever: it is the state of our minds, and that, and that alone, which is of importance. Therefore, ignoring entirely the illness from which we are suffering, we need consider only to which of the following types we belong.

Should any difficulty be found in selecting your own remedy, it will help to ask yourself which of the virtues you most admire in other people; or which of the failings is, in others, your pet aversion, for any fault of which we may still have left a trace and are especially attempting to eradicate, that is the one we most hate to see in other people. It is the way we are encouraged to wipe it out in ourselves.

We are all healers, and with love and sympathy in our natures we are also able to help anyone who really desires health. Seek for the out-standing mental conflict in the patient, give him the remedy that will assist him to overcome that particular fault, and all the encouragement and hope you can, then the healing virtue within him will of itself do all the rest.

NB As explained in the Foreword to this book, chapter XII of Free Thyself which describes the remedy types has been omitted because the description given represented Dr. Bach's earliest thoughts. For his complete and final work please refer to The Twelve Healers & Other Remedies which is available separately.

Ye Suffer
from Yourselves

By EDWARD BACH, *Physician,*
M.B., B.S., M.R.C.S., L.R.C.P., D.P.H.

Ye Suffer from Yourselves.

An address given at Southport, February, 1931.

IN coming to address you this evening, I find the task not an easy one.

You are a medical society, and I come to you as a medical man: yet the medicine of which one would speak is so far removed from the orthodox views of to-day, that there will be little in this paper which savours of the consulting room, nursing home, or hospital ward as we know them at present.

Were it not that you, as followers of Hahnemann, are already vastly in advance of those who preach the teachings of Galen, and the orthodox medicine of the last two thousand years, one would fear to speak at all.

But the teaching of your great Master and his followers has shed so much light upon the nature of disease, and opened up so much of the road which leads to correct healing, that I know you will be prepared to come with me further along that path, and see more of the glories of perfect health, and the true nature of disease and cure.

The inspiration given to Hahnemann brought a light to humanity in the darkness of materialism, when man had come to consider disease as a purely materialistic problem to be relieved and cured by materialistic means alone.

He, like Paracelsus, knew that if our spiritual and mental aspects were in harmony, illness could not exist: and he set out to find remedies which would treat our minds, and thus bring us peace and health.

Hahnemann made a great advance and carried us a long way along the road, but he had only the length of one life in which to work, and it is for us to continue his researches where he left off: to add more to the structure of perfect healing of which he laid the foundation, and so worthily began the building.

The homœopath has already dispensed with much of the unnecessary and unimportant aspects of orthodox medicine, but he has yet further to go. I know that you wish to look forward, for neither the knowledge of the past nor the present is sufficient for the seeker after truth.

Paracelsus and Hahnemann taught us not to pay too much attention to the details of disease, but to treat the personality, the inner man, realising that if our spiritual and mental natures were in harmony disease disappeared. That great foundation to their edifice is the fundamental teaching which must continue.

Hahnemann next saw how to bring about this harmony, and he found that among the drugs and the remedies of the old school, and among elements and plants which he himself selected, he could reverse their action by potentisation, so that the same substance which gave rise to poisonings and symptoms of disease, could – in the minutest quantity – cure those particular symptoms when prepared by his special method.

Thus formulated he the law of "like cures like": another great fundamental principle of life. And he left us to continue the building of the temple, the earlier plans of which had been disclosed to him.

And if we follow on this line of thought, the first great realisation which comes upon us is the truth that it is disease itself which is "like curing like": because disease is the result of wrong activity. It is the natural consequence of disharmony between our bodies and our Souls: it is "like curing like" because it is the very disease itself which hinders and prevents our carrying our wrong actions too far, and at the same time, is a lesson to teach us to correct our ways, and harmonise our lives with the dictates of our Soul.

Disease is the result of wrong thinking and wrong doing, and ceases when the act and thought are put in order. When the lesson of pain and suffering and distress is learnt, there is no further purpose in its presence, and it automatically disappears.

This is what Hahnemann incompletely saw as "like curing like".

COME A LITTLE FURTHER ALONG THE ROAD.

Another glorious view then opens out before us, and here we see that true healing can be obtained, not by wrong repelling wrong, but by right replacing wrong: good replacing evil: light replacing darkness.

Here we come to the understanding that we no longer fight disease with disease: no longer oppose illness with the products of illness: no longer attempt to drive out maladies with such substances that can cause them: but, on the contrary, to bring down the opposing virtue which will eliminate the fault.

And the pharmacopœia of the near future should contain only those remedies which have the power to bring down good, eliminating all those whose only quality is to resist evil.

True, hate may be conquered by a greater hate, but it can only be cured by love: cruelty may be prevented by a greater cruelty, but only eliminated when the qualities of sympathy and pity have developed: one fear may be lost and forgotten in the presence of a greater fear, but the real cure of all fear is perfect courage.

And so now, we of this school of medicine have to turn our attention to those beautiful remedies which have been Divinely placed in nature for our healing, amongst those beneficent, exquisite plants and herbs of the countryside.

It is obviously fundamentally wrong to say that ''like cures like.'' Hahnemann had a conception of the truth right enough, but expressed it incompletely. Like may strengthen like, like may repel like, but in the true healing sense like cannot cure like.

If you listen to the teachings of Krishna, Buddha, or Christ, you will find always the teachings of good overcoming evil. Christ taught us not to resist evil, to love our enemies, to bless those who persecute us – there is no like curing like in this. And so in true healing, and so in spiritual advancement, we must always seek good to drive out evil, love to conquer hate, and light to dispel darkness. Thus must we avoid all poisons, all harmful things, and use only the beneficent and beautiful.

No doubt Hahnemann, by his method of potentisation, endeavoured to turn wrong into right, poisons into virtues, but it is simpler to use the beauteous and virtuous remedies direct.

Healing, being above all materialistic things, and materialistic laws, Divine in its origin, is not bound by any of our conventions or ordinary standards. In this we have to raise our ideals, our thoughts, our aspirations, to those glorious and lofty realms taught and shown to us by the great Masters.

Do not think for one moment that one is detracting from Hahnemann's work, on the contrary, he pointed out the great fundamental laws, the basis; but he had only one life: and had he continued his work longer, no doubt he would have progressed along these lines. We are merely advancing his work, and carrying it to the next natural stage.

Let us now consider why medicine must so inevitably change. The science of the last two thousand years has regarded disease as a material factor which can be eliminated by material means: such, of course, is entirely wrong.

Disease of the body, as we know it, is a result, an end product, a final stage of something much deeper. Disease originates above the physical plane, nearer to the mental. It is entirely the result of a conflict between our spiritual and mortal selves. So long as these two are in harmony, we are in perfect health: but when there is discord, there follows what we know as disease.

Disease is solely and purely corrective: it is neither vindictive nor cruel: but it is the means adopted by our own Souls to point out to us our faults: to prevent our making greater errors: to hinder us from doing more harm: and to bring us back to that path of Truth and Light from which we should never have strayed.

Disease is, in reality, for our good, and is beneficent, though we should avoid it if we had but the correct understanding, combined with the desire to do right.

Whatever errors we make, it re-acts upon ourselves, causing us unhappiness, discomfort, or suffering, according to its nature. The object being to teach us the harmful effect of wrong action or thought: and, by its producing similar results upon ourselves, shows us how it causes distress to others, and is hence contrary to the Great and Divine Law of Love and Unity.

To the understanding physician, the disease itself points out the nature of the conflict. Perhaps this is best illustrated by giving you examples to bring home to you that no matter from what disease you may suffer, it is because there is disharmony between yourself and the Divinity within you, and that you are committing some fault, some error, which your Higher Self is attempting to correct.

Pain is the result of cruelty which causes pain to others, and may be mental or physical: but be sure that if you suffer pain, if you will but search yourselves you will find that some hard action or hard thought is present in your nature: remove this, and your pain will cease. If you suffer from stiffness of joint or limb, you can be equally certain that there is stiffness in your mind; that you are rigidly holding on to some idea, some principle, some convention may be, which you should not have. If you suffer from asthma, or difficulty in breathing, you are in some way stifling another personality; or from lack of courage to do right, smothering yourself. If you waste, it is because you are allowing someone to obstruct your own life-force from entering your body. Even the part of the body affected indicates the nature of the fault. The hand, failure or wrong in action: the foot, failure to assist others: the brain, lack of control: the heart, deficiency or excess, or wrong doing in the aspect of love: the eye, failure to see aright and comprehend the truth when placed before you. And so, exactly, may be worked out the reason and nature of an infirmity: the lesson required of the patient: and the necessary correction to be made.

Let us now glance, for a moment, at the hospital of the future.

It will be a sanctuary of peace, hope, and joy. No hurry: no noise: entirely devoid of all the terrifying apparatus and appliances of to-day: free from the smell of antiseptics and anæsthetics: devoid of everything that suggests illness and suffering. There will be no frequent taking of temperatures to disturb the patient's rest: no daily examinations with stethoscopes and tappings to impress upon the patient's mind the nature of his illness. No constant feeling of the pulse to suggest that the heart is beaing too rapidly. For all these things remove the very atmosphere of peace and calm that is so necessary for the patient to bring about his speedy recovery. Neither will there be any need for laboratories; for the minute and microscopic examination of detail will no longer matter when it is fully realised that it is the patient to be treated and not the disease.

The object of all institutions will be to have an atmosphere of peace, and of hope, of joy, and of faith. Everything will be done to encourage the patient to forget his illness; to strive for health; and at the same time to correct any fault in his nature;

and come to an understanding of the lesson which he has to learn.

Everything about the hospital of the future will be uplifting and beautiful, so that the patient will seek that refuge, not only to be relieved of his malady, but also to develop the desire to live a life more in harmony with the dictates of his Soul than had been previously done.

The hospital will be the mother of the sick; will take them up in her arms; soothe and comfort them; and bring them hope, faith and courage to overcome their difficulties.

The physician of to-morrow will realise that he of himself has no power to heal, but that if he dedicates his life to the service of his brother-men; to study human nature so that he may, in part, comprehend its meaning; to desire whole-heartedly to relieve suffering, and to surrender all for the help of the sick; then, through him may be sent knowledge to guide them, and the power of healing to relieve their pain. And even then, his power and ability to help will be in proportion to his intensity of desire and his willingness to serve. he will understand that health, like life, is of God, and God alone. That he and the remedies that he uses are merely instruments and agents in the Divine Plan to assist to bring the sufferer back to the path of the Divine Law.

He will have no interest in pathology or morbid anatomy; for his study will be that of health. It will not matter to him whether, for example, shortness of breath is caused by the tubercle baccillus, the streptococcus, or any other organism: but it will matter intensely to know what the patient is wrongly developing his love aspect. X-rays will no longer be called into use to examine an arthritic joint, but rather research into the patient's mentality to discover the stiffness in his mind.

The prognosis of disease will no longer depend on physical signs and symptoms, but on the ability of the patient to correct his fault and harmonise himself with his Spiritual Life.

The education of the physician will be a deep study of human nature; a great realisation of the pure and perfect: and an understanding of the Divine state of man: and the knowledge of how to assist those who suffer that they may harmonise their conduct with their Spiritual Self, so that they may bring concord and health to the personality.

He will have to be able, from the life and history of the

patient, to understand the conflict which is causing disease or disharmony between the body and Soul, and thus enable him to give the necessary advice and treatment for the relief of the sufferer.

He will also have to study Nature and Nature's Laws: be conversant with Her Healing Powers, that he may utilise these for the benefit and advantage of the patient.

The treatment of to-morrow will be essentially to bring four qualities to the patient.

First, peace: secondly, hope: thirdly, joy: and fourthly, faith.

And all the surroundings and attention will be to that end. To surround the patient with such an atmosphere of health and light as will encourage recovery. At the same time, the errors of the patient, having been diagnosed, will be pointed out, and assistance and encouragement given that they may be conquered.

In addition to this, those beautiful remedies, which have been Divinely enriched with healing powers, will be administered, to open up those channels to admit more of the light of the Soul, that the patient may be flooded with healing virtue.

The action of these remedies is to raise our vibrations and open up our channels for the reception of our Spiritual Self, to flood our natures with the particular virtue we need, and wash out from us the fault which is causing harm. They are able, like beautiful music, or any gloriously uplifting thing which gives us inspiration, to raise our very natures, and bring us nearer to our Souls: and by that very act, to bring us peace, and relieve our sufferings.

They cure, not by attacking disease, but by flooding our bodies with the beautiful vibrations of our Higher Nature, in the presence of which disease melts as snow in the sunshine.

And, finally, how they must change the attitude of the patient towards disease and health.

Gone forever must be the thought that relief may be obtained by the payment of gold or silver. Health, like life, is of Divine origin, and can only be obtained by Divine means. Money, luxury, travel, may outwardly appear to be able to purchase for us an improvement in our physical being: but these things can never give us true health.

The patient of tomorrow must understand that he, and he alone, can bring himself relief from suffering, though he may obtain advice and help from an elder brother who will assist him in his effort.

Health exists when there is perfect harmony between Soul and mind and body: and this harmony, and this harmony alone, must be attained before cure can be accomplished.

In the future there will be no pride in being ill: on the contrary, people will be as ashamed of sickness as they should be of crime.

And now I want to explain to you two conditions which are probably giving rise to more disease in this country than any other single cause: the great failings of our civilisation – greed and idolatory.

Disease, is, of course, sent to us as a correction. We bring it entirely upon ourselves: it is the result of our own wrong doing and wrong thinking. Can we but correct our faults and live in harmony with the Divine Plan, illness can never assail us.

In this, our civilisation, greed overshadows all. There is greed for wealth, for rank, for position, for worldly honours, for comfort, for popularity: yet it is not of these one would speak, because even they are, in comparison, harmless.

The worst of all is the greed to possess another individual. True, this is common amongst us that it has come to be looked upon as almost right and proper: yet that does not mitigate the evil: for, to desire possession or influence over another individual or personality, is to usurp the power of our Creator.

How many folk can you number amongst your friends or relations who are free? How many are there who are not bound or influenced or controlled by some other human being? How many are there who could say, that day by day, month by month, and year by year, "I obey only the dictates of my Soul, unmoved by the influence of other people?"

And yet, everyone of us is a free Soul, answerable only to God for our actions, aye, even our very thoughts.

Possibly the greatest lesson of life is to learn freedom. Freedom from circumstance, environment, other personalities, and most of all from ourselves: because until we are free we are unable fully to give and to serve our brother-men.

Remember that whether we suffer disease or hardship:

whether we are surrounded by relations or friends who may annoy us: whether we have to live amongst those who rule and dictate to us, who interfere with our plans and hamper our progress, it is of our own making: it is because there is still within us a trace left to bar the freedom of someone: or the absence of courage to claim our own individuality, our birthright.

The moment that we ourselves have given complete liberty to all around us: when we no longer desire to bind and limit: when we no longer expect anything from anyone: when our only thought is to give and give and never to take, that moment shall we find that we are free of all the world: our bonds will fall from us: our chains be broken: and for the first time in our lives shall we know the exquisite joy of perfect liberty. Freed from all human restraint, the willing and joyous servant of our Higher Self alone.

So greatly has the possessive power developed in the west that it is necessitating great disease before people will recognize the error and correct their ways: and according to the severity and type of or domination over another, so must we suffer as long as we continue to usurp a power which does not belong to man.

Absolute freedom is our birthright, and this we can only obtain when we grant that liberty to every living Soul who may come into our lives. For truly we reap as we sow, and truly ''as we mete so it shall be measured out to us.''

Exactly as we thwart another life, be it young or old, so must that re-act upon ourselves. If we limit their activities, we may find our bodies limited with stiffness: if, in addition, we cause them pain and suffering, we must be prepared to bear the same, until we have made amends: and there is no disease, even however severe, that may not be needed to check our actions and alter our ways.

To those of you who suffer at the hands of another, take courage; for it means that you have reached that stage of advancement when you are being taught to gain your freedom: and the very pain and suffering which you are bearing is teaching you how to correct your own fault, and as soon as you have realised the fault and put that right, your troubles are over.

The way to set about to do this work is to practise exquisite gentleness: never by thought or word or deed to hurt another.

Remember that all people are working out their own salvation; are going through life to learn those lessons for the perfection of their own Soul; and that they must do it for themselves: that they must gain their own experiences: learn the pitfalls of the world, and, of their own effort, find the pathway which leads to the mountain top. The most that we can do is, when we have a little more knowledge and experience than a younger brother, very gently to guide them. If they will listen, well and good: if not, we must patiently wait until they have had further experience to teach them their fault, and then they may come to us again.

We should strive to be so gentle, so quiet, so patiently helpful that we move among our fellow men more as a breath of air or a ray of sunshine: ever ready to help them when they ask: but never forcing them to our own views.

And I want now to tell you of another great hindrance to health, which is very, very common to-day, and one of the greatest obstacles that physicians encounter in their endeavour to heal. An obstacle which is a form of idolatory. Christ said "Ye cannot serve God and mammon," and yet the service of mammon is one of our greatest stumbling blocks.

There was an angel once, a glorious, magnificent angel, that appeared to St. John, and St. John fell in adoration and worshipped. But the Angel said to him, "See thou do it not, I am thy fellow servant and of thy brethren. Worship God." And yet to-day, tens of thousands of us worship not God, not even a mighty angel, but a fellow human being. I can assure you that one of the greatest difficulties which has to be overcome is a sufferer's worship of another mortal.

How common is the expression: "I must ask my father, my sister, my husband." What a tragedy. To think that a human Soul, developing his Divine evolution, should stop to ask permission of a fellow traveller. To whom does he imagine that he owes his origin, his being, his life – to a fellow-traveller or to his Creator?

We must understand that we are answerable for our actions, and for our thoughts to God, and to God alone. And that to be influenced, to obey the wishes, or consider the desires of another mortal is idolatory indeed. Its penalty is severe, it binds us with chains, it places us in prisons, it confines our very life; and so it should, and so we justly deserve, if we listen to the dictates of a human being, when our whole self should know but one command – that of our Creator, Who gave us our life and our understanding.

Be certain that the individual who considers above his duty his wife, his child, his father, or his friend, is an idolator, serving mammon and not God.

Remember the words of Christ, "Who is My mother, and who are My brethren," which imply that even all of us, small and insignificant as we may be, are here to serve our brother-men, humanity, the world at large, and never, for the briefest moment, to be under the dictates and commands of another human individual against those motives which we know to be our Soul's commands.

Be captains of your Souls, be masters of your fate (which means let your selves be ruled and guided entirely, without let or hindrance from person or circumstance, by the Divinity within you), ever living in accordance with the laws of, and answerable only to the God Who gave you your life.

And yet, one more point to bring before your notice. Ever remember the injunction which Christ gave to His disciples, "Resist not evil." Sickness and wrong are not to be conquered by direct fighting, but by replacing them by good. Darkness is removed by light, not by greater darkness: hate by love: cruelty by sympathy and pity: and disease by health.

Our whole object is to realise our faults, and endeavour so to develop the opposing virtue that the fault will disappear from us like snow melts in the sunshine. Don't fight your worries: don't struggle with your disease: don't grapple with your infirmities: rather forget them in concentrating on the development of the virtue you require.

And so now, in summing up, we can see the mighty part that homœopathy is going to play in the conquest of disease in the future.

Now that we have come to the understanding that disease itself is "like curing like": that it is of our own making: for our correction and for our ultimate good: and that we can avoid it, if we will but learn the lessons needed, and correct our faults before the severer lesson of suffering is necessary. This is the natural continuation of Hahnemann's great work; the sequence of that line of thought which was disclosed to him, leading us a step further towards perfect understanding of disease and health, and is the stage to bridge the gap between where he left us and the dawn of that day when humanity will have reached that state of advancement when it can receive direct the glory of Divine Healing.

The understanding physician, selecting well his remedies from the beneficent plants in nature, those Divinely enriched and blessed, will be enabled to assist his patients to open up those channels which allow greater communion between Soul and body, and thus the development of the virtues needed to wipe away the faults. This brings to mankind the hope of real health combined with mental and spiritual advance.

For the patients, it will be necessary that they are prepared to face the truth, that disease is entirely and only due to faults within themselves, just as the wages of sin is death. They will have to have the desire to correct those faults, to live a better and more useful life, and to realise that healing depends on their own effort, though they may go to the physician for guidance and assistance in their trouble.

Health can be no more obtained by payment of gold than a child can purchase his education: no sum of money can teach the pupil to write, he must learn of himself, guided by an experienced teacher. And so it is with health.

There are the two great commandments: "Love God and thy neighbour." Let us develop our individuality that we may obtain complete freedom to serve the Divinity within ourselves, and that Divinity alone: and give unto all others their absolute freedom, and serve them as much as lies within our power, according to the dictates of our Souls, ever remembering that as our own liberty increases, so grows our freedom and ability to serve our fellow-men.

Thus we have to face the fact that disease is entirely of our own making, and that the only cure is to correct our faults. All true healing aims at assisting the patient to put his Soul and mind and body in harmony. This can only be done by himself, though advice and help by an expert brother may greatly assist him.

As Hahnemann laid down, all healing which is not from within, is harmful, and apparent cure of the body obtained through materialistic methods, obtained only through the action of others, without self-help, may certainly bring physical relief, but harm to our Higher Natures, for the lesson has remained unlearnt, and the fault has not been eradicated.

It is terrible to-day to think of the amount of artificial and superficial cures obtained through money and wrong methods in medicine; wrong methods because they merely suppress symptoms, give apparent relief, without removing the cause.

Healing must come from within outselves, by acknowledging and correcting our faults, and harmonising our being with the Divine Plan. And as the Creator, in His mercy, has placed certain Divinely enriched herbs to assist us to our victory, let us seek out these and use them to the best of our ability, to help us climb the mountain of our evolution, until the day when we shall reach the summit of perfection.

Hahnemann had realised the truth of "like curing like," which is in reality disease curing wrong action: that true healing is one stage higher than this: love and all its attributes driving out wrong.

That in correct healing nothing must be used which relieves the patient of his own responsibility: but such means only must be adopted which help him to overcome his faults.

That we now know that certain remedies in the homœopathic pharmacopœia have the power to elevate our vibrations, thus bringing more union between our mortal and Spiritual self, and effecting the cure by greater harmony thus produced.

And finally, that it is our work to purify the pharmacopœia, and to add to it new remedies until it contains only those which are beneficent and uplifting.

Part Two

Readers will be interested to note from the following correspondence with the C. W. Daniel Company that "Heal Thyself" was originally called "Come out into the Sunshine", but as this title implied that the subject matter may be connected with "sunshine therapy", the book was re-named.

The first royalty statement is also illustrated here as a point of interest. The £7 12s 10d received would, in those days, have gone a long way and helped a great deal to fund the work. Still today, royalties are put towards future publications of the books to help maintain prices at an affordable level.

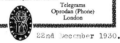

THE C. W. DANIEL COMPANY
(C. W. DANIEL, D. M. WALTHAM)

46 Bernard Street, London, W.C.1
(Opposite Russell Square Tube Station)

Telephone
Terminus
4691

Telegrams
Oprodan (Phone)
London

22nd December 1930.

Dr. Edward Bach
4, St.Marys Road
Cromer
Norfolk.

Dear Sir,

We have read with very great interest and pleasure the
typescripts of your work "COME OUT INTO THE SUNSHINE".   Implicit
throughout its pages is the unsullied desire for the physical health
and spiritual well-being of humanity, which places it as a work
worthy to be published.   At the same time that very character takes
it beyond the bounds of ordinary commercial venturing.

We have had experience in marketting books of a similar character.
For,instance, "THE DIVINE ART OF HEALING", an old medical essay
by Dr.Hahnemann, a veritable classic.   And yet such is the materialism
of our time that such a work, worthy to sell by the tens of thousands,
is insignificant in relation to sales compared with works which,
however commendable from the standpoint of materia medica, are from
the point of view of spiritual healing and psycho-therapeutics, are
inadequate.

Frankly, we should like to publish your work if it were possible
for us to do so without our having to take the full financial responsibility.   It would interest us to know, therefore, whether you would
consider a proposal whereby both parties shared the costs of publication
and the proceeds of sales.

Yours faithfully

THE C. W. DANIEL COMPANY
CW Daniel

4, St. Mary's Road,
Cromer,
Norfolk.

December 24.1930.

Dear Sirs,

Re " Come out into the sunshine."

May I thank you very much
indeed for your courteous letter.
I fully realise the diffic-
-ulty of publication, and the uncertainty
of a market, though being fairly well known
in the medical and a certain social world,
there would be ~~a certain~~ some demand in that
direction.
~~benefit~~ I have no desire to ~~have~~ Receive
any financial ~~interest~~ in the sale of this
small work, it is one of those things one
wishes to give, and I would also be pleased
to pay a portion of the expense of produc-
-tion, ~~if you~~ will you kindly let me know the
amount,(and if it is within my means, which
are unfortunately limited,) I will send
you a cheque without delay.

Yours sincerely,

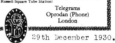

THE C. W. DANIEL COMPANY
(C. W. DANIEL, D. M. WALTHAM)

46 Bernard Street, London, W.C.1
(Opposite Russell Square Tube Station)

Telephone
Terminus
4691

Telegrams
Oprodan (Phone)
London

29th December 1930.

Dr. Edward Bach
4, St.Marys Road
Cromer
Norfolk.

Dear Sir,

We write to acknowledge receipt of your letter of December 24th., and to say that we hope this further letter may enable you to decide whether we are to co-operate with you for the publication of "COME OUT INTO THE SUNSHINE".

We were prepared at the first sight of the typescript of your work to consider it as coming definitely within the scope of medical or health literature. In which case your name and degrees would have counted heavily on the side of its being a full risk book for a publisher. As it is there is danger that the title and your degrees may lead readers to suppose that it is a book as we supposed it to be, viz:, on Sunlight Therapy. And that leads us to ask whether it would not be better to choose another title or add to the present an explanatory sub-title. It is a question, of course, which may be settled leisurely during the time taken for the type-setting of the book.

We enclose a copy of a small book which we propose as model for your own - excepting that the number of pages would be about 16 pages more.

The total cost of manufacturing 1000 copies similar to sample would be £80. We propose, therefore, that you should contribute £40 which would be refunded out of sales at the rate of 1/2 per copy i.e 50% of the sale proceeds which would be two-thirds of the published price (published price 3/6). On further editions called for we should accept full financial responsibility and pay a royalty of 15% of the published price on 12 out of every 13 copies sold.

Yours sincerely,

TH. C.W.DANIEL COMPANY

CWDaniel

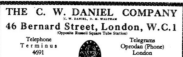

THE C. W. DANIEL COMPANY
[C. W. DANIEL, D. M. WALTHAM]

46 Bernard Street, London, W.C.1
(Opposite Russell Square Tube Station)

Telephone
Terminus
4691

Telegrams
Oprodan (Phone)
London

1st January 1931.

Dr. Edward Bach
4, St.Mary's Road
Cromer
Norfolk.

Dear Sir,

We write to thank you for your letter of December 31st., covering cheque for £40 and we value the confidence so freely given to us. It will be as well to implement the contract by a formal document. We will therefore send in the course of two or three days a stamped and signed agreement, (which will act also as a receipt for £40) and a copy for your signature and return.

We have given your typescripts with necessary instructions to our printers who will, we believe, start sending in proofs about the end of next week. They will first be read by us and then sent to you.

Provisionally, we may fix the date of publication as February 26th. It may be possible to publish before then but it is customary for us to guarantee publication within 60 days of the execution of agreement.

The third paragraph of your letter serves as excellent descriptive matter for use on the book's dust jacket. We should choose "HEAL THYSELF" for the title and, for sub-title, "An Explanation of the Real Cause and Cure of Disease". We do not like the use of the word "fundamental" in a title and we should seek to avoid using "real" with "reason". The following is our redraft of the paragraph referred to :-

Dr. Bach shows what are the vital principles which will guide medicine in the near future and are indeed guiding some of the more advanced members of the profession today. His book therefore comes directly into the practical politics of medicine.

It is perfectly certain we shall not regret the association with your book. Having put our hands to the plough we shall not look back.

Yours sincerely,
THE C.W.DANIEL COMPANY

73

THE C · W · DANIEL COMPANY

(C. W. Daniel and D. M. Waltham)

Telephone
Central
7611

PUBLISHERS

Telegrams
Oprodan, Phone
London

46 ~~E~~ ~~XXXXXXXX~~ STREET, LONDON, ~~XXXX~~ W.C.1.
BERNARD

No 3321   *December 31* 1932

M. *Dr E. Bach*

Statement of Sales of " *Heal Thyself* "

Edition			588
	on sale		12
Copies Free (Review Copies, etc.)			
„ Sold		131	
„ on Hand		469	
„ on Sale		600	600

Royalty Account

By Royalties on Sales			
131 @ 1/2	£ 7	12 10	

Part Three

The following is a collection of philosophical notes written by Dr. Bach on April 22nd 1933, whilst staying in Marlow, Buckinghamshire. His words never fail to instil hope and re-awaken one's faith in Life.

Marlow, Bucks
April 22 1933

In main principle, the fault on earth is the desire for worldly things: a great danger in heaven is the greed and too great desire for spiritual things: and just as on earth greed can so hamper the rising soul, you will find the same in spiritual life, where utter humility and service is needed rather than the desire for perfection.

The desire to be good, the desire to be God, may be as great a hindrance in spiritual life as the desire for gold or power is in earthly experience. The further one advances the greater must be the humility and the patience and the desire to serve.

In the old path, you were fighting the greed for gold (gold is the emblem of worldly power); in the new world, strange though it may seem, you are fighting the greed for good. 'Which of us should be greater in the Kingdom of Heaven'.

The hindrance to spiritual advance, is the desire to progress. In this Kingdom it is 'being', not aspiring: the 'being' brings its own reward. This refers not only to this life, but more so to those who seek the spiritual world. There must be no desire to be good, no desire for rapid improvement or perfection, but to be humbly content to wait in any station of service until called to a higher.

In this Realm, we do not progress by our own effort, but merely wait until we are considered worthy.

On earth, effort: in Heaven, the reverse.

This means that to make even the greatest sacrifice on earth for the sake of gaining spiritual greatness, even this is wrong. It is like the rich young man who said 'All these have I done', but it did not open to him the door of heaven.

It seems as though the only way is impersonal service, done, not even for spiritual promotion, but just only the desire to serve. This is the keynote of the hindrances you are now to investigate.

We are used to training ourselves that our bodies must not count, that there must be no self: then must be realised that our souls must not count.

For the next coming of Christ, there is a band of people who, to welcome Him, should be able to transcend their physical natures and realise their spirituality.

Man has so come to look upon the body as himself, that it is difficult for him to know that it is but an instrument. He has even taken the teaching of re-incarnation in the wrong way, because instead of that convincing him of his immortality and the unimportance of a body, he, instead, becomes a little proud of his several lives, and what he has been and what he has done.

Life on earth is but a thing of darkness in comparison with spiritual life, and in it the truth can rarely be seen. How like a chicken in the shell being proud of itself, so proud, so self-important in its isolation that it refused to break its way out, and would rather die in its darkness. 'Tis very largely the fear of losing individuality that prevents man accepting spiritual truth; but like the chicken in the shell, he does not lose himself by going out into the world of light.

The world today is full of people who fear to break the shell of self-importance, and thus remain prisoners in their tiny world. Fear of loss of self is behind this, and this prevents all growth, all gaining of real knowledge.

It is no use in the present time just to say 'Don't be afraid', or, 'Don't be ill'. It is necessary to tell them why they are afraid, why they are ill, and to give them the antedote.

Just as has been shown to us the reasons of illness, and the herbs divinely placed for our use to correct our faults and heal our bodies, so now is it necessary to learn how to show people why they are afraid and the remedy which lies within themselves how to overcome fear.

Physical illness is a material thing: fear is mental. The former can be dealt with by physical means of a very high order. And just as the herbs have an uplifting power on the body and the mind, so the next healing prepares the mind for spiritual union and conscious governing of the life by the Divinity within.

Essentially it is greed that is the origin of physical disease, and fear of mental.

In this Realm there is no faith, no hope, no doubt, it is CERTAINTY. Time is of no account, space matters not.

Seek and watch that you miss no opportunity of learning that you may be able to help others, for after you have sought and watched in the world, in quiet moments will come the answer to your problem from within yourself.

You do not settle up your difficulties in the world, but after study of your surroundings and careful quiet thought, you prepare yourself for the enlightenment which comes from within. Knowledge sought to aid one to help others earns, so to speak, your right to that knowledge: and whilst in the world you should very quietly persevere and watch and seek without tiring.

The inner knowledge comes to you without effort in unexpected moments of peace or repose or when the mind is employed on other things. 'Seek and ye shall find'.

Ye seek with your senses and your mind, but the answer comes from your soul within. It is thus the swallows learnt to fly across the ocean.

Part Four

Dr. Bach would often write about the remedies as though they were personalities in their own right. Here are some examples – stories of the Centaury, Clematis and Oak.

One of the favourites – "The Story of the Travellers" – is included in *The Bach Flower Remedies Step by Step* by Judy Howard, and therefore not repeated here.

September 1933.

The Story of Clematis itself.

CLEMATIS.

And do you wonder that I want to go away? You see, I have fixed my thoughts on earthly things, on earthly people, and if they go I so want to follow them. I just want to fly away and be where they are. Can you blame me? My dreams, my ideal, my romance. Why should I not be with all these things, and what can you offer me that is better? Nothing that I can see. You only offer me cold materialism, life on the earth with all its hardships and sorrows, and there far-away is my dream, my ideal. Do you blame me if I follow it?

And Clematis came along and said, 'Are your ideals God's ideals? Are you sure that you are serving Him Who made you, Who created you, Who gave you your life, or are you listening just to some other human being who is trying to claim you, and so you are forgetting that you are a son of God with all His Divinity within your soul, and instead of this glorious reality you are being lured away by just some other human being.

I know how we long to fly away to more wonderful realms, but, brothers of the human world, let us first fulfill our duty and even not our duty but our joy, and may you adorn the places where you live and strive to make them beautiful as I endeavour to make the hedges glorious, so that they have called me the 'Travellers' Joy'.

September 1933.

The Story of Centaury itself.

CENTAURY.

I am weak, yes, I know I am weak, but why? Because I have learnt to hate strength and power and dominion, and if I do err a little on the weakness side, forgive me, because it is only a reaction to the hatred of hurting others, and I shall soon learn to understand how to find the balance when I neither hurt nor am hurting. But just for the moment I would rather that I suffered than that I caused one moment's pain to my brother.

So be very patient with your little Centaury, she is weak, I know, but it is a weakness on the right side, and I shall soon grow bigger and stronger and more beautiful until you will all admire me because of the strength I shall bring to you.

The Story of the Oak Tree.

———————

One day, and not very long ago, a man was leaning against an oak tree in an old park in Surrey, and he heard what the oak tree was thinking. Now that sounds a very funny thing, but trees do think, you know, and some people can understand what they are thinking.

This old oak tree, and it was a very old oak tree, was saying to itself, 'How I envy those cows in the meadow that can walk about the field, and here I am; and everything around so beautiful, so wonderful, the sunshine and the breezes and the rain, and yet I am rooted to the spot.'

And years afterwards the man found that in the oak flowers of the oak tree was a great power, the power to heal a lot of sick people, and so he collected the flowers of the oak trees and made them into medicines, and lots and lots of people were healed and made well again.

Some time after this on a hot summer's afternoon, the man was lying on the edge of a corn-field very nearly asleep, and he heard a tree thinking, as some people can hear trees think. The tree was speaking to itself very quietly, and it was saying, 'I don't any longer mind being rooted to the spot, and I don't any longer envy the cows who can walk about the meadows, because I can go to all the four quarters of the world to heal the people who are ill': and the man looked up and found it was an oak tree thinking.

Part Five

The following pages contain a collection of letters – some to journals, others to friends and colleagues.

It will interest readers to note that the first of these letters referred to the link between the remedies and astrology. Dr. Bach held this subject in high regard but did not wish to adopt it as a means of prescribing as it did not allow for the finer considerations of mood and outlook which are so important when selecting the most appropriate remedies.

In one letter, dated November 15th 1933, you will note Dr. Bach's last line "have started journeying, so far so good". He had, by that time, found another four remedies to complement his original twelve, and as always, he wasted no time in bringing them to the notice of the public. In August 1933 he wrote a small pamphlet describing these four remedies and soon afterwards had his work formally published in a booklet called "The Twelve Healers and the Four Helpers".

After a while, he found a further three remedies and so had his work re-published, with a new title – "The Twelve Healers and the Seven Helpers". The title "Twelve Healers" was retained throughout because Dr. Bach felt it had become familiar to those who knew his work.

October 9. 1933.

    Dear Wheeler,

                Good to you for your series of
cases in Heal Thyself.
                I don't feel inclined personally
to send Barker any more contributions. He is dis-
-gruntled because he is unable to use the remedies
himself, and from the way the magazine is going
the question arises whether he is doing Homoeopathy
any good. Is he not leading his audience further
and further away from mentals?
                We may later get persecution from
this quarter, but even so it will help us.
                He has so repeatedly demanded from
us pathological readings of the remedies (which
of course are impossible to give), and I know is
annoyed that he has not been able to get them.
                We must watch his lordship care-
-fully lest he be an opponent instead of a friend
to the whole homoeopathic science.

                Congratulations on your mastoid
case, and we do admire your courage.

            All the very best of wishes,

                        Edward Bach.

*Your letter about mastoid just arrived.
Splendid my friend. good to you.
and so it can be with all acutes.
Most grateful for all your encouragement.*

4. Brunswick Terrace.
Cromer.
Norfolk.

October 29. 1933.

Dear Folk,

Enclosed what I feel to be two very wonderful papers, they are not very long but they con--tain an immense ground work of thought. Miss Weeks' paper also is very fitting to these three.
If you approve of all we are sending you we are certainly keeping you stocked well ahead.
I am being very cautious as regards astrology, and that is why one left out the Signs and the months in the first Twelve Healers. This work is decidedly going to assist vastly in the purifica--tion and understanding of astrology, but my part seems to be to give general principles whereby people like you who have a more detailed knowledge, may dis--cover a great truth. That is why I do not wish to be associated with anything dogmatic, until one is sure.
The enclosed one knows is right, and hence ready for publication, but the exact placing of Signs and planets and bodily systems, for the moment, has not certainty.

With the very best of wishes to you,

Edward Bach.

Might these three appear in same magazine.? merely suggestion.

4. Brunswich Terrace,
Cromer.
Norfolk.

Dear Folk.

I think Miss Weeks'
article is the simplist and
most beautiful yet written.
She is a mighty power for
good: because childlike she
sees things from the simple pure
way. T'any rate that's
how it strikes me: see what
you think.
Our love to you:
Brave comrades.

The fourth contribution to
complete the series.

May they find satisfaction
in your eyes. !

More to follow from Miss Weeks
before long.

You hit a wonderful good point
when you say: not necessary to
wait for physical diagnoses and
so save time. yes! very often
life.   The best of wishes.

                                   4, Brunswick Terrace,

                                      Cromer.

November I5. I933.

        Dear Folk,

                Wouldn't it be just as well to put the year of treatment.
or else the duration of the cure afterwards with the cases recorded
in the magazine to show that they are not all cases of just the pres-
-ent.

        As regards case 3 of the Agrimony cases. The patient has now
worked hard and kept well for three years. She was first treated
in I930.
        As regards case 4. Although life has still been difficult for
this patient, he has remained in good health and a much better mental
state for the last three years. Treated I930.
        As regards cases5. No further news of this patient since I930.

                Again very much like Mrs Wheeler's article. One tiny
suggestion. Does not Agrimony open the door to let in the golden vital
breath of peace. One always feels that the light of Agrimony is so
very closely associated with 'the peace that passeth understanding',
the peace of the Christ; whilst the love is more that glorious blue,
that of Chicory, to my mind the nearest earthly colour which one
associates surrounding our Lady, His Mother.
                If any such suggestions interrupt Mrs Wheeler's train
of thought, tell me to shut up.

                Will bear dedicatory article in mind. Hope to let you
have it shortly, don't quite yet know what to say.

                Have started journeyings, so far so good.

                All the very best of wishes,

                                    Edward Bach.

instead
of love.

4, Brunswick Terrace,
Cromer,
Norfolk.

December 5.1933.

The sort of letter that gives us encouragement. A case of SCLERANTHUS. A man who was in a very bad way, and through loss of all self-confidence was desperate.

"Dear Sir,

It is with the greatest pleasure I am writing this letter to you, to tell you that the medicine which you prescribed for me is doing me a world of good.

I am gradually beginning to regain my old confidence and in a few weeks will be completely cured. I can honestly say you have done me more good in two weeks than five London doctors have done in three years, amongst whom is Doctor——————, head of the Hospital for ——————————,
————————.

Once again, Doctor, I wish to say, I thank you for your great kindness in sending me those prescriptions, and I will write again to let you know when I am completely cured."

4, Brunswick Terrace,
Cromer,
Norfolk.

January 17.1934.

Dear Brother,
This was the beginning of our Four Helpers.

One day, feeling anxious as regards the future, as I suppose we are all liable to do at times, I was lying near the tow-path at Marlow-on-Thames, when this message came through. A message not only for myself, but for all those who are striving to help.

I wrote it down as it is, and instantly noticed by my side a gorse bush in full bloom, and I thought 'How beautiful'. I had not seen it before, but then I thought of the wondrous sight of moorlands covered with the flaming bush.

This was the first of our Four Helpers.

I got up and went straight to a woman I knew about, self-centred and utterly worldly, and I said to her, 'What do you think is the most beautiful sight in the world? Have you ever seen anything that makes you think it possible that there is a God?' Without the least hesitation she replied, 'Yes, the mountains covered with heather'.

And so was found the second of our Helpers.

To many people, of course, this would mean nothing, but to you, I know, it shows the way by which the White Brotherhood work, amongst us, not by miracles, not by apparitions, but just leading us, if we are willing to be led, by every-day affairs.

EDWARD BACH

Part Six

Dr. Bach met Nora Weeks shortly before he left London, and he invited her to accompany him on his travels. She felt deeply privileged because she respected his compassion and dedication enormously, believing unconditionally in his endeavour. She took great pleasure in painting locations where he first found a particular remedy, and a few of these paintings are included here for your interest. Dr. Bach would also jot down the places where he found the remedy plants in his copy of "British Wild Flowers" by J.E. Sowerby & C.P. Johnson but as he loved all of nature's wild flowers, he would make a note of each one that he came across on his travels. You will see from the excerpt of this book, and the following map which emphasises the areas visited, that his journey took him far and wide!

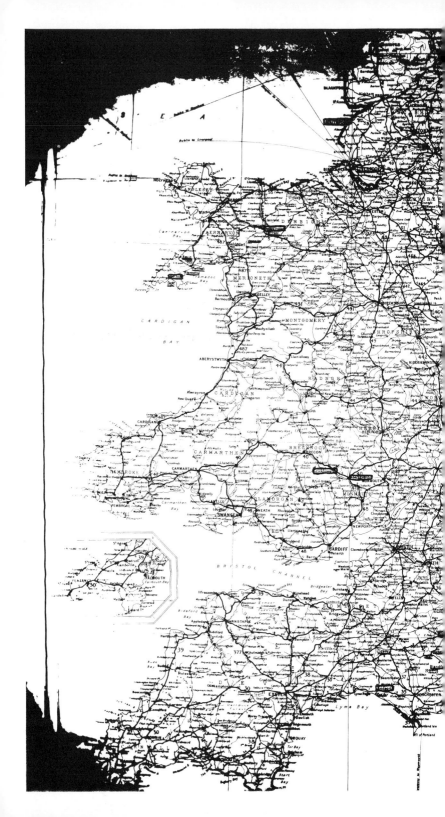

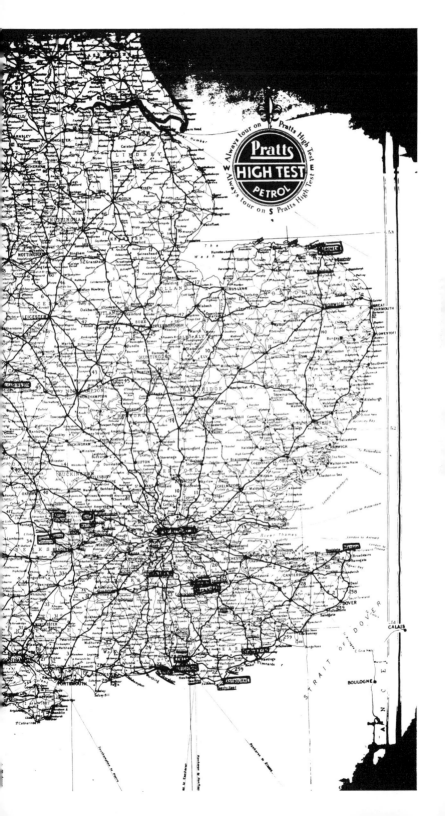

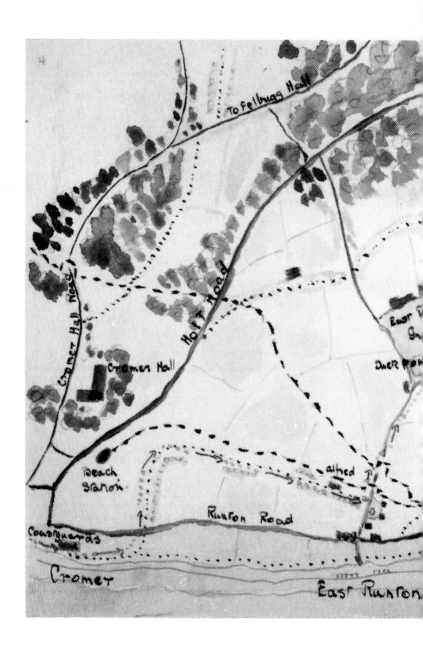

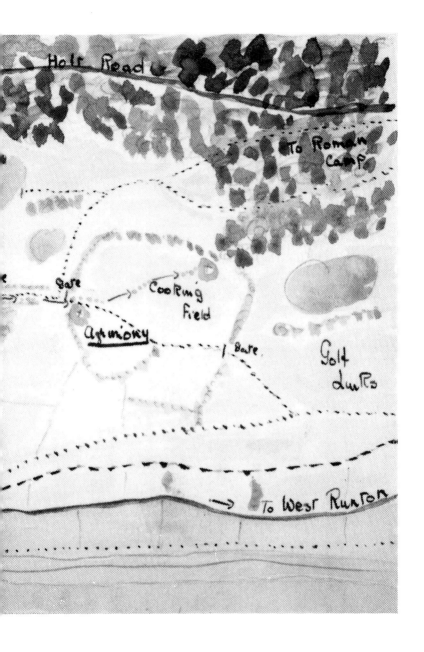

Impatiens

ROAD

Marsh

Mimulus.

+

cooking
Field.

RAPIDS

RIVER Uck.

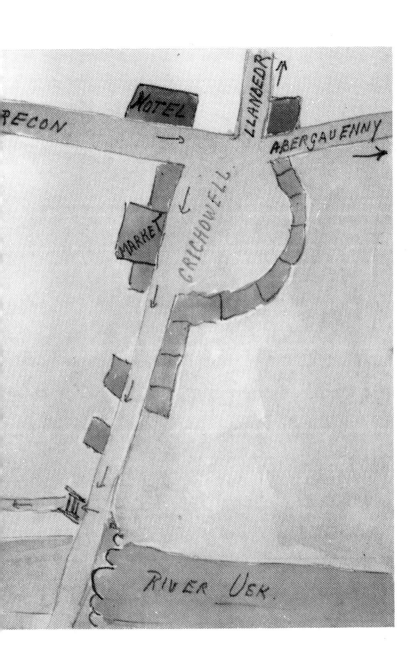

BRECON
NOTEL
LLANBEDR
ABERGAUENNY
CRICHOWELL
MARKET
RIVER USK.

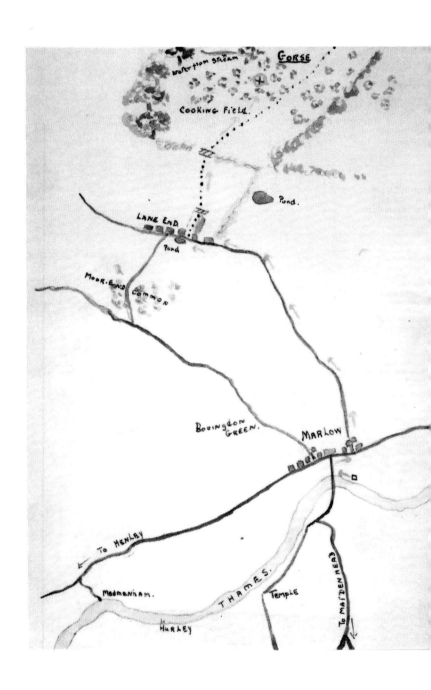

GORSE

Water from Stream

Cooking Field

Pond.

LANE END

Pond

MOOR END

COMMON

BOVINGDON GREEN.

MARLOW

TO HENLEY

Medmenham.

THAMES.

Temple

HURLEY

TO MAIDEN HEAD

ORDER XL. LORANTHACEÆ.
Genus 1. VISCUM.

V. ALBUM. *Mistletoe.* **Fig. 581.**
A parasitic shrub. Stems forked. Leaves opposite. Diœcious. On apple and other trees. March–May. Yellowish; berries white. ($\frac{2}{3}$) *E. B.* 1. 1470. *E. B.* 2. 1386. *H. & Arn.* 191. *Bab.* 153. *Lind.* 133.

ORDER XLI. CAPRIFOLIACEÆ.
Genus 1. SAMBUCUS.

S. EBULUS. *Dwarf Elder. Dane-wort.* **Fig. 582.**
Leaflets lanceolate. Stem herbaceous. Cymes with 3 branches. Waste ground. Violently purgative. 2–3 ft. Perenn. July. Pink; berries black. ($\frac{2}{3}$) *E. B.* 1. 475. *E. B.* 2. 444. *H. & Arn.* 192. *Bab.* 154. *Lind.* 132.

S. NIGRA. *Common Elder.* **Fig. 583.**
A large shrub. Leaflets ovate. Cymes with 5 principal branches. Hedges; common. Bark and leaves cathartic. 8–15 ft. June. White; berries black. ($\frac{2}{3}$) *E. B.* 1. 476. *E. B.* 2. 445. *H. & Arn.* 192. *Bab.* 154. *Lind.* 132.

Genus 2. VIBURNUM.

V. LANTANA. *Meal-tree.* **Fig. 584.**
A shrub. Leaves heart-shaped, serrated, downy beneath. Hedges and thickets. 6–12 ft. June. White; berries purple when ripe. ($\frac{2}{3}$) *E. B.* 1. 331. *E. B.* 2. 442. *H. & Arn.* 193. *Bab.* 154. *Lind.* 132.

V. OPULUS. *Guelder Rose.* **Fig. 585.**
A large shrub. Leaves 3-lobed, serrated. Outer flowers barren, with one large 5-lobed petal. Woods. 10–15 ft. June. White; berries red. ($\frac{2}{3}$) *E. B.* 1. 332. *E. B.* 2. 443. *H. & Arn.* 193. *Bab.* 154. *Lind.* 132.

Genus 3. LONICERA.

L. CAPRIFOLIUM. *Perfoliate Honeysuckle.* **Fig. 586.**
A climbing shrub. Upper leaves united round the stem. Woods; rare. May and June. White or purple. ($\frac{2}{3}$) *E. B.* 1. 799. *E. B.* 2. 324. *H. & Arn.* 193. *Bab.* 154. *Lind.* 131.

L. PERICLYMENUM. *Honeysuckle. Woodbine.* **Fig. 587.**
A climbing shrub. Leaves separate. Flowers in terminal heads. Woods; common. June and July. Pale yellow, red outside. ($\frac{2}{3}$) *E. B.* 1. 800. *E. B.* 2. 325. *H. & Arn.* 193. *Bab.* 154. *Lind.* 131.

L. XYLOSTEUM. *Upright Honeysuckle.* **Fig. 588.**
A shrub. Flower-stalks 2-flowered. Thickets in Sussex. June. Pale yellow. ($\frac{2}{3}$) *E. B.* 1. 916. *E. B.* 2. 326. *H. & Arn.* 193. *Bab.* 155. *Lind.* 132.

Genus 4. LINNÆA.

L. BOREALIS. **Fig. 589.**
A small creeping shrub. Leaves opposite. Flowers in pairs, drooping. Northern Pine-woods. 6–8 in. Perenn. May and June. White or pale rose-colour. ($\frac{2}{3}$) *E. B.* 1. 433. *E. B.* 2. 884. *H. & Arn.* 194. *Bab.* 155. *Lind.* 132.

ORDER XLII. RUBIACEÆ.
Genus 1. RUBIA.

R. PEREGRINA. *Wild Madder.* **Fig. 590.**
Leaves 4 in a whorl, oval, with prickles on the margin, evergreen. Shady thickets. 8 in. Perenn. July. White. ($\frac{2}{3}$) *E. B.* 1. 851. *E. B.* 2. 218. *H. & Arn.* 195. *Bab.* 159. *Lind.* 131.

I 2

Genus 4. SALICORNIA.

Abersoch. *June. 30*

S. HERBACEA. *Glasswort.* **Fig. 1041**
Stem erect. Lower branches compound. Spikes cylindrical. Salt marshes and muddy shores. 6–10 in. Ann. Aug. Yellowish green. ($\frac{2}{3}$) *E. B.* 1. 415. *E. B.* 2. 1. *H. & Arn.* 360. *Bab.* 278. *Lind.* 214.

S. PROCUMBENS. *Procumbent Glasswort.* **Fig. 1042.**
Stem procumbent. Branches simple. Spikes tapering. A variety of *herbacea.* Salt marshes. 6 in. Ann. Aug. Yellowish green. ($\frac{2}{3}$) *E. B.* 1. 2475. *E. B.* 2. 1*. *H. & Arn.* 360. *Bab.* 278. *Lind.* 214.

S. RADICANS. *Creeping Glasswort.* **Fig. 1043.**
Stems woody, rooting at the base. Joints compressed. Spikes oblong. Muddy sea-shores. 1 ft. Perenn. Aug. Yellowish green. ($\frac{2}{3}$) *E. B.* 1. 1691. *E. B.* 2. 2. *H. & Arn.* 360. *Bab.* 278. *Lind.* 214.

S. FRUTICOSA. *Shrubby Glasswort.* **Fig. 1044.**
Stems woody. Joints cylindrical. Spikes cylindrical. A variety of *radicans.* 1 ft. Perenn. Aug. Yellowish green. ($\frac{2}{3}$) *E. B.* 1. 2467. *E. B.* 2. 2*. *H. & Arn.* 360. *Bab.* 278. *Lind.* 214.

Genus 5. SALSOLA.

Gromer. *Soft. 33.*

S. KALI. *Saltwort.* **Fig. 1045.**
Stems procumbent. Leaves awl-shaped, spine-pointed. Calyx with a membranous expansion. Coasts. 1 ft. Ann. July. Pinkish. ($\frac{2}{3}$) *E. B.* 1. 634. *E. B.* 2. 364. *H. & Arn.* 362. *Bab.* 275. *Lind.* 214.

ORDER LXX. SCLERANTHACEÆ.

Genus 1. SCLERANTHUS.

Bryslÿd + Chael/ *r/ 1/y.32*

S. ANNUUS. *Knawel.* **Fig. 1046.**
Stems many, procumbent. Calyx of fruit with erect or spreading segments. Corn-fields; common. 4–6 in. Ann. July. Green. ($\frac{2}{3}$) *E. B.* 1. 351. *E. B.* 2. 591. *H. & Arn.* 362. *Bab.* 125. *Lind.* 218.

Gromer. *Soft. 30.*

S. PERENNIS. *Perennial Knawel.* **Fig. 1047.**
Calyx of fruit with incurved segments, edged with a white membrane. Sandy fields. 4 in. Perenn.? Aug.–Nov. Green. ($\frac{2}{3}$) *E. B.* 1. 352. *E. B.* 2. 590. *H. & Arn.* 363. *Bab.* 125. *Lind.* 218.

ORDER LXXI. POLYGONACEÆ.

Genus 1. POLYGONUM.

P. BISTORTA. *Bistort. Snakeweed.* **Fig. 1048.**
Stem simple, bearing one spike. Leaves ovate, waved; the lower ones with a winged foot-stalk. Moist meadows. Root very astringent. 1–1$\frac{1}{2}$ ft. Perenn. June–Sept. Pale pink. ($\frac{2}{3}$) *E. B.* 1. 509. *E. B.* 2. 571. *H. & Arn.* 363. *Bab.* 283. *Lind.* 212.

P. VIVIPARUM. *Alpine Bistort.* **Fig. 1049.**
Stem bearing one spike. Leaves linear-lanceolate, with revolute margins. Lower buds of the spike viviparous. Mountain pastures. 6 in. Perenn. July. Pale pink. ($\frac{2}{3}$) *E. B.* 1. 669. *E. B.* 2. 572. *H. & Arn.* 364. *Bab.* 283. *Lind.* 212.

Abersoch *June. 30*

P. AVICULARE. *Knot-grass.* **Fig. 1050.**
Stem procumbent. Leaves elliptic-lanceolate. Flowers axillary. Fruit rough and striated, covered by the calyx. A common weed. 1–6 in. Ann. April–Nov. Pinkish. ($\frac{2}{3}$) *E. B.* 1. 1253. *E. B.* 2. 573. *H. & Arn.* 364. *Bab.* 285. *Lind.* 212

P

CHAPTER III

THE FINAL YEARS – 1934–1936

Part One

Having discovered nineteen remedies, an account of which had been published in "The Twelve Healers and the Seven Helpers", Dr. Bach felt that it was time to settle down. He chose the Thames Valley as he liked the area and knew it well. He had always wanted to live by a river in a quiet village surrounded by open countryside, so the village of Sotwell tucked away at the foot of the Chiltern Hills with the River Thames within talking distance, was an ideal retreat. It was not long before a little house called Mount Vernon, set in the heart of Sotwell, became his home.

Dr. Bach soon had a team of helpers to assist him with his work. Nora Weeks who had been with him throughout, Victor Bullen whom he met in Cromer, and a lady from the village of Sotwell, Mary Tabor. Miss Tabor lived at a house called Wellsprings which was a much larger house than Mount Vernon, and so Dr. Bach would sometimes work from there, hence the appearance of that address on some of his letters.

It was during the latter two years of his life, spent at Sotwell, that he discovered the last nineteen remedies to complete his discovery of the 38 flowers. He would often send samples of plants to the Royal Botanic Gardens at Kew for identification and confirmation of species so that he could describe them accurately.

Dr. Bach was extremely excited by his new findings. It was as though, at last, the final pieces of the jigsaw were fitting together, and his joyous mood is clearly reflected in his letters at that time.

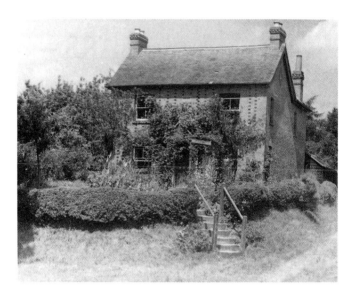

*A very early photograph of 'Mount Vernon',
Dr. Bach's home from 1934–1936.*

ROYAL   BOTANIC   GARDENS,

KEW,   SURREY.

25th June, 1934.

D. 2736

Dear Sir,

In reply to your letter of the 22nd
June, the grass forwarded for identification
is Bromus ramosus Huds.

Yours faithfully,

Arthur Hill

Director.

Dr. Edward Bach,
        Mount Vernon,
                Sotwell,
                        Wallingford,
                                Berks.

Mount Vernon,

Sotwell,

Wallingford,

BERKS.

July 1

Dear Friends,

The prescription of these new remedies is going
to be much more simple than at first appeared, because each of
them corresponds to one of the Twelve Healers or the Seven
Helpers.

For example: supposing a case is definitely
Clematis and does fairly well but not a complete cure, give the
corresponding new remedy further to help the cure.

Enclosed a list of those already worked out;
the rest we shall receive in due time.

There is not doubt that these new remedies act on
a different plane to the old. They are more spiritualized and
help us to develop that inner great self in all of us which has
the power to overcome all fears, all difficulties, all worries,
all diseases.

We may know more of this difference later on,
but in all of us, whilst there are definite earthly fears of
which we are so very conscious, there are also those vague un-
-known fears which are more frightening than those of material
things; and there is no doubt that in all of those of us who
strive to help our fellow men, who strive to do a little good on
our journey through the world, those unknown fears are more
common.

Edward Bach.

August 4.1935.
Sotwell.

No man would be a leader amongst others for any length of time unless he were more expert in his special branch of knowledge than his followers: whether it be army, statesmanship or whatever it may be.

It therefore follows, to be a leader against trouble, difficulties, disease, persecution and so forth, the leader must still have a greater knowledge, a more intimate experience than, pray God, his followers need ever suffer.

EDWARD BACH

a

WELLSPRINGS,
SOTWELL,
WALLINGFORD,
BERKS.

September 24. 1935.

Dear Brother Doctor Wheeler,

What a splendid case of Aspen.
Thank you so very much for the report.

The more we use these remedies,
both the new nineteen and the old nineteen,
the more wonderful the results; and the
people who know of them ▮ have such faith
that they can be cured, no longer come
and say 'Can you put me right', but just
expect it and take it for granted.

Very kindest wishes to you from
all of us.

Edward Bach.

I have not yet quite thought out the
table you sent, but hoping to let you
have a reply about this quite shortly.

WELLSPRINGS.
SOTWELL.
WALLINGFORD.
BERKS.

September 25.1935.

Dear Friends,

If any of us were arranging a picnic or a party next Wednesday, we should all hope for fine weather, and if any of us were responsible for the arrangements, we might go through a few days' fear and anxiety as to whether it would be fine or not. Some of us would have, perhaps, a few days of real unhappiness.

But if we knew that next Wednesday was going to be wet or fine, we should either alter the day or make arrangements to suit the conditions, and there would be no anxiety or fear or unhappiness.

And so it must be with all our fears. It is the ignorance that lies behind: and this seems to be our next problem to remove the ignorance and KNOW.

The life-boat men have no fear because they know they will safely return, or if, as very rarely happens, they are drowned, they know that all is well.

Fear in some way attracts the very thing of which we are afraid. We bring it upon ourselves. To KNOW would save the fear, or in other words to quote, 'Ye shall know the TRUTH, and the TRUTH shall make you free'.

Our next problem, all of us, is to KNOW; and each of us in our own way, and any one of us, may be the one to find the solution.

The two cases of which some of you know about, prove so strongly how lack of knowledge causes fear.

The one man, terrified to go in a train, always asked the engine-driver if the communication cord was in order, tested the door handles to see if they opened easily, tested emergency doors of motor buses, and suffered much. The moment he realised he was doing all this in the public interest, for the sake of his fellow-passengers, and that he would be the last man to leave any wreck, all the load and dread of travelling went out of his mind, and it was extraordinary how much happier he became.

The other man who studied science for upwards of forty years, had expert knowledge of almost every branch, had been researching to prove everything could be accounted for by a material explanation. He was unhappy, argumentative and miserable because he found missing links in all directions. But the moment he realised that his life's work had been spent to prove behind it all there was a God, his whole life changed; and as a great scientist no one is more capable or more ardent to continue his mission in the right direction.

These two cases ilustrate what is happening to so many of us, and it would turn our arduous and difficult lives into lives of joy if we KNEW instead of always fearing.

So we can know that those of us who have fear are doing good work. It is only just we do not realise that our own fear is for the good of others.

The great secret seems to be – to be afraid and not to be afraid of being afraid, until the time comes when we realise that we are right and are doing good.

Certainty, knowledge, truth would remove from our minds all fear, yet it may be part of the Divine Plan we prove ourselves far greater by battling on, though we are afraid; and it is for mankind to discover the way to see the Light and remove from mankind the burden of fear.

The wonderful remedies that we have, especially MIMULUS for physical fears, and especially ASPEN for mental fears, by the marvellous help they give to suffering people, must have been placed for our use by Divine Providence.

In this little centre, our little group, the results of healing by the Herbs are daily proving so wonderful, and we can say daily, that we, and it seems it is no exaggeration to say, that hundreds around us, have completely lost all fear of disease. No matter what greek or latin or French or English name it carries we know, and it has been proved in all around that all fear of illness is disappearing.

This is a step in the right direction.

May the Great Creator of all help us all to further His Work, until all fears, all anxieties are replaced by childlike naturalness and joy of living.

EDWARD BACH

Wellsprings,
Sotwell,
Wallingford,
BERKS.
December 26.1935.

Dear Brothers all,
The whole essence of life is to KNOW our Divinity; that we are unconquerable, invincible, and that no hurt can ever stop us in the victory which we are winning in the Name of our Great Master.
And for folk like ourselves who think of others, who wish to serve, who devote so much of our time and of our worldly good to those in need, could there be any other reason that we do this unless we knew within ourselves that we are
DIVINE.

Let us take this Truth in both hands and go forward unafraid. Have we ever wanted for a roof or a crust of bread and cheese? Have we ever wanted for far greater luxuries than these?
Let us all walk Ladies and Gentlemen Unafraid; ever bearing in mind one of the last messages given to us by our Master,
'LO! I AM WITH YOU ALWAYS'.

EDWARD BACH

Part Two

As Dr. Bach's work of healing with the Flower Remedies became more well-known, word spread and people would flock to Mount Vernon for treatment. We still have Dr. Bach's case histories, his prescription note books and original mother tinctures at the Centre.

You will notice from the examples of some of his cases included here, that although physical complaints are mentioned (which are, of course, natural considerations for a doctor), the remedies chosen for the patient have, in each case, been prescribed in accordance with the mood and personality. The number of remedies chosen at any one time varies with the individual needs – for some, only one or two were needed, for others five or six, and on some occasions eight or nine remedies were required.

Miss Breedon.

Crab Apple. Impatiens. Star Bett.
Mimulus. Aspen. Cherry Plum.
Rock Rose. Agrimony. Sweet Chestnut.

Mr Michael Meers.
                    wwman   eyes. hereditary

Chicory. Walnut. Mimulus. Aspen.
Red Chestnut.

Miss Mountford   Secretary
Centaury Mustard Honeysuckle Clematis
Agrimony Walnut Scleranthus Oak
Cerato.

Miss Burchill (Oales) **14.**

Rock Water
Water Violet.

? Scleranthus

big soul

58.

MRS Allcock.

1933. Sciatica.

July. 10   Smf.

12   Smf. Ag.

13   Smf. Ag.

                        +

17.   Gorse + Impatiens

18.   Mimp. Scl. Smf.

20   GORSE.

20   Water Violet   Smf.   Vervain.

21ˢᵗ   Water Violet   Imp.   Vervain +

23ʳᵈ   "   "   "   "

24ᵗʰ   "   "   "   "   pain in leg some

25ᵗʰ   "   "   "   "

26ᵗʰ   Agrimony.

27   Agrimony + Gentian.   back a little better.

28   Agrimony + Gentian

29ᵗʰ   Oak + Scleranthus.

31   GORSE.

Aug. 2.   R. Rose. Mim. Ag. +
                    pain in back less

Aug. 4th   Gorse. R. Rose. Mim. Agrimony.
Aug. 8th   Clem. Sel. Gent. Chicory.

"   Ag. Smp. + Clematal I

" 10   Ag. + Imp —
" 11.   Ag. Imp. Clem. Seler.
" 15.   Rock Water —
" 17.   Rock Water. +
" 24th   Rock Water.
" 30th   Rock Water + Gorse + +.
Sept. 4th Rock Water + Gorse
" 8th   R. Water. Mim. Imp.
   11.   Gentian. Smp. + Med. V
" 14th   Gentian. Imp.
" 15.   Vervain. Smp.
" 18th   Heather Impatiens.
" 20th   Heather Impatiens R. Water.
" 27.   Cerato. Centaury. Mimulus. Gentian
" 30th   Cerato. Centaury.

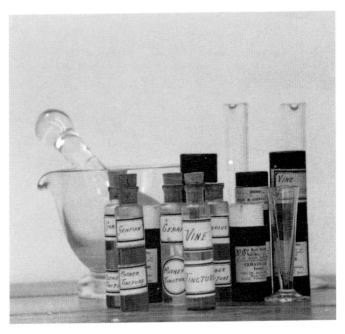

Dr. Bach's original mother tinctures.

THE REMEDIES AT WORK

The following cases, illustrating the use of Clematis, are taken from Dr. Bach's Case-Books:

1. *Male. Age 37.*

HISTORY.

Sent by a firm in which he held responsible position and was a valuable servant, because for the last few months he had become indifferent to his work and was quite unconcerned as to his failure to fulfil his obligations. His wife died one year ago.

PRESENT STATE.

Always sleepy; great difficulty in waking in the morning; continually feeling that he had lost confidence and ability to continue his work. Loss of power to concentrate. Perfectly complacent and obviously paying no real interest in present day affairs, his mind being concerned with other matters.

DIAGNOSIS.

The utter complacency to failure, lack of effort and dreamy apathy indicate Clematis.

DOSAGE.

1930. Nov. 7. Two doses for two days.
       Nov. 24. Two doses for two days.
1931. Jan. 2. Two doses for one day.

PROGRESS.

There has been steady, gradual improvement, and the patient has been able to continue work with increasing efficiency. He is now considered to have reached his normal state. The last six weeks an urticarial rash has been occurring and is definitely associated with the improvement.

———————

2. *Male. Age 47.*

HISTORY.

Overworked in city for several years. Last three months almost complete loss of memory; at times unable to remember home address or telephone number. Becomes sleepy during the day and indifferent to his work. Domestic tragedy seven years ago.

PRESENT STATE.

Expression vacant; thoroughly apathetic; quite contentedly resigned to the fact that he has become useless, making no effort for cure. Only with difficulty persuaded by friends to seek medical advice.

DIAGNOSIS.

The drowsy state, the apathy, absence of all interest, and resignation, denote Clematis.

DOSAGE.

1930. May 1. Two doses.
Sept. 4. Two doses.

PROGRESS.

Rapid improvement followed; the patient resumed business and worked well until the end of August, when there was some relapse, and more doses were given. Since then, the patient has remained well and in a recent letter stated that he considered himself cured.

———————

3. *Female. Age 38.*

HISTORY.

Asthma all life. Seven years ago lost favourite daughter; since then became an invalid. Six years ago, right arm and leg became paralysed, with difficuty of speech. This followed the birth of a son and was probably due to cerebral thrombosis. The patient was unconscious for three weeks at the time.

PRESENT STATE.

Moderate chronic asthma. Right arm completely paralysed, hanging by side, all sensation absent. Right leg spastic; able to walk with difficulty; very rigid. Speech hardly understandable, except to family.

CHARACTER.

Patient obviously living in dreams; unable to concentrate or give any fixed attention; continually weeping over the loss of her daughter.

DIAGNOSIS.

The dreamy state, the complete living in the past and the absence of interest in the present, indicated Clematis.

DOSAGE.

Nov. 24. Two doses for two days.
Dec. 1. Two doses for two days.

PROGRESS.

No sign of asthma since the first dose. There is a complete return of interest in daily life, and every effort is being made to get well. All sad memories of the past have disappeared. The speech is quite understandable to strangers. There is less spasticity in the leg with more natural and easy movement; the patient has walked five miles without undue fatigue. A return of power, sensation and movement has begun in the right arm and hand.

She is full of happiness and joyful excitement at every little improvement and is steadily progressing.

———

Burns due to electric shock.

4. *Male. Age 21.*

This was a case of unusual interest, which illustrates the use of the remedies both internally and externally.

HISTORY.

The patient was engaged in erecting electric cables, and at the time of the accident was working at the top of a thirty foot pole. He was dealing with a "live" wire, and while working on it the wind blew the "earth" cable against him and so made contact with his body. He received the 700 volts through him; his right hand, which was clutching the "live" wire, clenched round it, and, as is usual when a strong current passes through the body, he was unable to let go. The earth wire being removed from him, he fell thirty feet on to a hedge below, thus breaking his fall. He was picked up in a semi-conscious condition.

TREATMENT.

Oct 24. Four days later, the patient was seen by me. The right hand was swollen to about three times its normal size; severe and deep burns were present on the ball of the thumb, between the ring and little finger and also on the outer side of the hand. The hand was devoid of all sensation and in a sense was "dead"; there was complete absence of pain.

Clematis was given internally to bring back life into the hand. Impatiens was added to a lotion to act as a balm to the wounds.

Oct. 26. The hand now began to come to life, as it were, being sensitive to touch over the back of it, and was now painful if allowed to hang down. The swelling also was less. During the morning, the patient accidentally trod on a pet dog, and the yelp it gave caused him to jump up and then sit down "trembling and shivering all over", just as he had done after receiving the electric shock. The patient was outwardly cheerful and making light of his injuries.

Agrimony, Mimulus and Rock Rose were given internally; Agrimony for the mental state of cheerfulness in spite of his injury, Mimulus to soothe the nervous system, and Rock Rose to ward off possible complications, such as haemorrhage from the wounds.

Oct. 28. Hand much less swollen, but inclined to be painful when dressed; slight bleeding for the first time from the burn wounds.

Impatiens was added to the Calendula lotion used to dress the hand; Impatiens and Agrimony were given internally, Impatiens for the pain and Agrimony, as before, for the mental outlook.

Oct. 30. The wounds, which so far had shown very little healthy reaction, now became somewhat offensive, especially over the ball of the thumb area, and the hand now required dressing twice daily. Two of the fingers were shaking and trembling. The patient was not "himself", not yet "back" as it were, after the shock he had received. No feeling or sensation in the thumb or in the ball of it yet. Hand now almost normal size.

Scleranthus, Clematis and Gentian given internally: Scleranthus for the unsteadiness of the fingers, Clematis to bring the patient back, and Gentian as there was some depression.

Nov. 2. Improving, but still some insensitiveness of thumb and surrounding area.

Nov. 5. A certain amount of trembling of the hand, when trying to open and shut the fingers.

Clematis, Gentian and Scleranthus given internally; Clematis to bring back "life", Scleranthus for the trembling, and Gentian for some slight depression still remaining.

Nov. 11. Going on well, except for some stiffness of the fingers, particularly of the thumb, which was quite locked.

Vervain given internally and also added to the lotion, in order to combat the stiffness.

Nov. 17. Hand much better; could do some typing with his fingers; wounds practically closed, except for the very large one on the ball of the thumb, where the tissues had been charred down to the fascia.

Vervain given for some slight remaining stiffness, and Impatiens was used in the dressings in case the nerves should cause pain.

Nov. 18. When the patient came for the next dressing, not only could the thumb be moved quite freely, but he said he was wonderful; felt uncommonly fit and was able to take a ten mile walk.

From this day onwards there was rapid improvement; the large wound closed without further discharge, and new skin formed naturally. It became evident that there would be no need for skin-grafting, and that neither would there be any disability left in the hand. Very little scarring was left, and that only over the ball of the thumb, where the burn had been of the fourth degree.

———————

You will have noticed in the foregoing case histories, that certain states of mind seemed prevalent, yet no mention was made of remedies we would recognize as being appropriate. The reason for this is that the treatment of these cases took place BEFORE Dr. Bach had completed his work, hence the slight discrepancies.

If we were dealing with Case No. 4 today, we would most certainly have applied Rescue Remedy Cream to the wound. This, however, was formulated much later, but it would, nevertheless, be interesting to know how beneficial it might have been if Dr. Bach had it available to him then!

Part Three

Having proved through their use that the remedies were of great value, Dr. Bach was dismayed at the attitude taken by his Profession. He received numerous letters from the General Medical Council questioning his activities, the status of his helpers, and the newspaper advertisements he had placed to inform people of the new system of healing. After a long series of correspondence between the G.M.C. and Dr. Bach, he was ultimately told to stop his activities or risk his name being struck off the register. But Dr. Bach was so convinced and certain of the benefit of his new work that he would not be detracted from his convictions. The duty of a doctor, he maintained, was to heal the sick and relieve their suffering, and his replies to the Council's letters reflected his feelings to this effect.

Dr. Bach's name was never removed from the Register.

AN APPEAL.

To my Colleagues of the Medical Profession.

After very many years of research, I have found that certain Herbs have the most wonderful healing properties; and that with the aid of these, a large number of cases which by orthodox treatment we could only palliate, are now curable.

Moreover, on-coming disease can be treated and prevented at that stage when people say, 'It is not bad enough to send for a doctor'.

But when we gain the confidence of those around that disease should be tackled in its very earliest stages, and moreover, when we are able to explain to them that in the most obstinate and chronic cases it is worth while persevering with treatment, our work will be widely extended. Because we shall have that army of people come to us, days, weeks or months before they otherwise would to have their health adjusted; and secondly, the chronic cases will not only send for us when they wish for relief of pain or discomfort, but will send to us to continue with their cases in the hopes of a cure being obtained.

The Herbs mentioned can be used in conjunction with any orthodox treatment, or added to any prescription, and will hasten and assist the treatment in all types of cases, acute or chronic, to be more successful.

It is a time amongst us when orthodox medicine is not fully coping with a proportion of disease in this country; and it is a time to regain the confidence of the people, and justify our noble Calling.

The Herbs are simple to every student of human nature to understand, and one of their properties is that they help us to prevent the onset of organic disease when the patient is in that functional state which, in either acute or chronic ailments, so often precedes them.

Wellsprings,
Sotwell,
Wallingford, BERKS.
January 8.1936.

To the President of the General Medical Council.
Dear Sir,
Having received the notification of the Council concerning working with unqualified assistants, it is only honourable to inform you that I am working with several, and shall continue to do so.

As I have previously informed the Council, I consider it the duty and privilege of any physician to teach the sick and others how to heal themselves. I leave it entirely to your discretion as to the course you take.

Having proved that the Herbs of the field are so simple to use and so wonderfully effective in their healing power, I deserted Orthodox medicine.

Registered medical address.
Berryfields,
Park Lane,
Ashstead,
Surrey.

Wellsprings,
Sotwell,
Wallingford,
Berks.
January 8.1935.

Dear Brothers,
Enclosed a copy of a letter sent today to the General Medical Council, which will very shortly prohibit any of our Team by law from visiting houses.

The sick will have to come to us, or parents or relatives report to us the nature of the case.

This we know is very right, as it is those who make an effort who get well.

It is the kind of people who took up a flooring because the throng was so great that it was the only way to reach a Healer.

EDWARD BACH.

Part Four

The following is a selection of papers written by Dr. Bach during his last years. Many of you may remember excerpts which have, from time to time, been included in the Bach Remedy Newsletter.

LET US BE OURSELVES.

Has it ever occurred to you that God gave you an individuality? Yet He certainly did. He gave you a personality of your very own, a treasure to be kept to your very own self. He gave you a life to lead, which you and only you should lead: He gave you work to do, which you and only you can do: He placed you in this world, a Divine being, a child of Himself, to learn how to become perfect, to gain all knowledge possible, to grow gentle and kind, and to be a help to others.

And has it ever occurred to you how God speaks to you, and tells you of your own individuality, and of your very own work, of how to steer your ship true to its own course? He speaks to you through your own real desires which are the instincts of your Soul. How else could He speak?

If we but listen to and obey our own desires, uninfluenced by any other personality, we shall always be led aright; we shall always be guided, not only along the path which will lead us to our own advancement and perfection, but also to make our lives to the uttermost useful and helpful to others. It is being influenced by the desires of others that takes us from our own work and wastes our time. Christ would never have fulfilled His Mission had He listened to the persuasion of his parents, and we should have lost an army of world-helpers such as Florence Nightingale and a host of others, had they yielded to the wishes of others and not remained true to their own heart's desires.

What better resolution in the coming of the New year can we make than to listen to our own desires which are messengers from our Souls, and to have the courage to obey them.

TWO MORE ESSENTIALS

By Dr. E. Bach

There are two essentials that the healer must ever bear in mind when helping a patient. The first is to encourage their individuality, and the second to teach them to look ahead.

Once we are really our own true individuality, our own personality, when we have learnt: "To thine own self be true", disease cannot inflict itself upon us. Once the soul and mind and body are in harmony, illness is past.

In these days of convention many find it difficult to be themselves and yet it can be done.

Every human being is unique, in that he or she has a personality of their very own, which should not be swamped in the flood of the modern tendency to destroy character, which strives to make us just units or numbers or parts of a great machine. Every single person has a life to live, a work to do, a glorious personality, a wonderful individuality, if they will but realise it, and if they can hold this and keep this against all the laws of conforming to the mass, they will shine out and help others as examples of character.

Throughout the ages, those who have remained true unto themselves have ever been looked upon as men and women of genius, for in whatever station they have been placed, they have fulfilled their destiny. The world loves those and is inspired by those who have the courage and the indifference towards public opinion to carry out their mission. And everyone should be an example of individuality.

The healer should recognise in the sick that their malady is due to the loss of spiritual expression which follows the cramping of their Divine mission by the thoughts and influences of those around.

Then the other point, to look ahead or to look forward.

Most mountaineers, most steeple-jacks, most captains of ships will tell you to look ahead, to look in front of you or to look above you, but not to look behind or below. And so with our patients. Never let them for one moment think of the past; that is over and done with, and no matter what the faults, the mistakes, the slips, let these be forgotten and banished from the mind, for the past will have taught its lesson, and this will have been imprinted deeply enough without reminder. It is the view ahead, the glimpse of the above, that will stimulate and encourage them and bring them the hope to struggle on. As the mountaineer looks to the summit which he hopes to attain, so in life they must earnestly and constantly keep their eyes fixed on the glorious future and never court depression by looking backwards. All their mistakes, their slips, their faults of the past have been merely experiences to teach them better, to show them the right way from the wrong; in their souls that lesson has been well learnt, and they should not burden their minds by thinking back of what they might consider failures, for no matter how big the slips they may have made in climbing the mountain, no matter what wrongs they may have done or how terrible they may appear to them, these were merely experiences sent to them for their education and, having been experienced, may be forgotten, as the lesson will live in them. All that they should think is that it was a necessity to help them upwards and a blessing in disguise.

For these reasons never allow patients to talk about the past. The illness of yesterday is of yesterday, and of no interest or importance now. What we have to treat is the present state of the patient, exactly as he is at the time we see him, and even when we see him again in a further week, he is again a new patient. Improvements may have occurred and alterations taken place, which now mean that he may require another remedy, and even the interval of a week gone by is past history and of no present consequence. In acute cases our patient may be a new man, a different case within a few hours. We must ever treat the present NOW, and to think back or to allow a patient to dwell on the past is hampering in its results.

No matter how serious the illness, no matter what right or wrong may have occurred in the past, it is the hope of the future, of better and more glorious times ahead that will spur the invalid to victory.

Thus teach people, as children of the Creator, the Divine individuality within them which is able to overcome all trials and difficulties; help them to steer their ship over the sea of life, keeping a true course and heeding not others; and teach them also ever to look ahead, for, however they may have gone out of their course and whatever storms and tempests they may have experienced, there is always ahead for everyone the harbour of peace and security.

———————

May 21.1936

All TRUE KNOWLEDGE comes ONLY from WITHIN OURSELVES, in silent communication with your own Soul.

Doctrines and civilisation have robbed us of the Silence, have robbed us of the Knowledge that WE KNOW ALL WITHIN OURSELVES.

We have been led to believe that we must be taught by others, and our own Spiritual Selves have become SUBMERGED.

The acorn, carried hundreds of miles from it's mother-tree, knows without instruction how to become a perfect Oak. The fish of the sea and rivers lay their spawn and swim away. The same with the frog. The serpent lays it's eggs in the sand, and goes on it's journey; and yet within the acorn, and the spawn, and the eggs is all the knowledge necessary for the young to become as perfect as their parents.

Young swallows can find their way to their Winter quarters hundreds of miles away, whilst parent birds are still busy with the second brood.

We need so much to come back to the knowledge that WITHIN OURSELVES LIES ALL TRUTH. To remember that we need seek no advice, no teaching but from within.

The Christ taught us that the lilies of the field, though they neither toiled nor spun, were more perfectly arrayed than Solomon in all his glory.

And the Lord Buddha taught us that we were well on the path to our SELF REALISATION once we became rid of the priests and the books.

13.12.33

What we call 'love' is a combination of greed and hate, that is, desire for more and fearing to lose. Therefore what we call 'love' must be IGNORANCE.

Real love must be infinitely above our ordinary comprehension, something tremendous, the utter forgetfulness of self, the losing of the individuality in the Unity, the absorption of the personality in the Whole.

Thus it appears that love is the very opposite of self.

When we understand these terms then shall we understand the teachings of Christ, they will no longer be parables. Love, in a way, seems to be service combined with wisdom.

What we call 'love' is everyone who gives to us because it satisfies our desire of greed for more, and what we call hate is everyone who takes from us because it stimulates our fear of losing.

When we realise that we have nothing on this earth that is not worth while losing, but everything to gain, then we cannot know hate and then in the proper meaning of the word we shall be able to 'love our enemies'.

Real love of God or our fellows seems to be the desire to serve without reward.

Probably the nearest we ever know to love is for the unattainable, sunsets, starry nights, music, and the beauty of the mountains and moors.

In our heart of hearts we must know that our enemies are those who give way to us, because by so doing they make a bond, a bond we find almost impossible to break and we thank them when they struggle free.

Anyone over whom we can influence our will or control or power is a danger to our freedom. No matter whether our influence is due to love or power or fear or what they get from us. Our Souls must thank all those who refuse to be our servants, since it robs both them and us of our individuality.

––––––––––––

CHAPTER IV

Conclusion of The Work

Part One

As soon as Dr. Bach knew that the thirty-eight remedies covered every negative state of mind and that there were no more to find, he announced his work to be complete, and immediately began, as was his custom, to re-write his findings in a final book which he called "The Twelve Healers & Other Remedies".

He then destroyed all his old notes, pamphlets and books – even his photographs! – be means of a bonfire in the garden at Mount Vernon. Nora and Victor were "horrified" to see so much profound work turned to ashes, but Dr. Bach explained that his work had now reached its conclusion, the last edition of the Twelve Healers being the final and complete record of his discovery. All that led to it – his research work and the previous editions of his book – were, he said, superfluous and potentially misleading, and in an effort to protect readers from unnecessary confusion, he burnt everything.

Thankfully, some of his papers and a photograph escaped the bonfire, and among them, the following correspondence between Dr. Bach and his publisher, regarding the ultimate edition of the Twelve Healers. You will see from this that they too were requested to destroy all previous editions! So although we do have copies of these books, we have, with respect for his wishes, not re-printed them because we do not wish to detract from the purity of his final findings.

Shortly before he died, in November 1936, Dr. Bach wrote an extended introduction to the book and asked that it be included in the next edition. Nora Weeks made sure this wish was granted, but it was not until 1941 that the next edition was due for publication. Since then, the book has been reprinted seventeen times!

THE C. W. DANIEL COMPANY
(C. W. DANIEL, D. M. WALTHAM)
46 Bernard Street, London, W.C.1
(Opposite Russell Square Tube Station)

Telephone
T e r m i n u s
4691

Telegrams
Oprodan (Phone)
London

24th July 1936

Ref. CWD/M.

Dr. Edward Bach
Wellsprings,
Sotwell,
Wallingford,
Berks.

Dear Sir,

We have received your letter of July 19th and have considered your decision to entirely revise and extend your book "THE TWELVE HEALERS". While we regret the necessity to destroy so much as at least half the present edition, we admire very much your desire in the interest of healing work to present to the public your new findings.

We think the price of such special work, if it is to be enlarged, should also be increased.

We will undertake to publish without any consideration of cash payment by you. Costs can be recovered out of sale proceeds. Should you be in a position at any time to provide a fund for advertising in special papers, we think that should tend to increase the sales.

At present there are about 900 copies in stock.

Yours sincerely

THE C.W.DANIEL COMPANY LTD

Ref. CWD/M.

July 25.1936.

Messrs Daniels.

Dear Sirs,

Many thanks for your letter of the 24th. Am very pleased to know that you will undertake publication of the third edition of 'The Twelve Healers'. And thank you very much indeed for your offer to recover cost out of sale proceeds.

This edition, I hope, and expect will remain the permanent one.

Enclosed under separate cover, manuscript complete in every detail for printing.

Will you please get this on the market as soon as possible and in due course destroy all copies of the present edition.

Definite interest is being taken in this work in America, and we are promised funds from that quarter, part of which could certainly be expended in advertising.

Yours sincerely,

EDWARD BACH.

THE C. W. DANIEL COMPANY
(C. W. DANIEL, D. M. WALTHAM)
46 Bernard Street, London, W.C.1
(Opposite Russell Square Tube Station)

Telephone
Terminus
4691

Telegrams
Oprodan (Phone)
London

31st July 1936

REF. CWD/M.

Dr. Edward Bach,
Wellsprings,
Sotwell,
Wallingford,
Berks.

Dear Sir,

Third Edition, "THE TWELVE HEALERS"

We were pleased to receive the note re title, which
we have added to Introduction. "Wild Oat" has been
uniformly put on pages 9 and 32. Rock Water has been
added to the list of names at end and the place for the
Latin equivalent left blank.

We have also taken the liberty of adding to your
additional note to Introduction the following: "The
original twelve are indicated by asterisks" We have
added the asterisks to the names in the Remedies Section
and in the list of names.

The typescripts are now with the Printers and you
will receive proofs by August 13th or 14th.

Yours faithfully

THE C.W. DANIEL COMPANY LTD.

[signature]

August 1.1936.

Messrs Daniel.

Re Third Edition 'The Twelve Healers'

Dear Sirs,
      If the sum of five pounds would be of sufficient value to assist in advertising the third edition of "The Twelve Healers", we can place that amount at your disposal in about ten days' time.
      This is not in connection with the fund I mentioned, which has not yet materialised.

      Yours sincerely,

EDWARD BACH

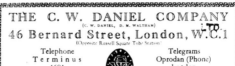

THE C. W. DANIEL COMPANY LTD

(C. W. DANIEL, D. M. WALTHAM)

46 Bernard Street, London, W.C.1

(Opposite Russell Square Tube Station)

Telephone
Terminus
4691

Telegrams
Oprodan (Phone)
London

2nd September 1936

Ref. CWD/M

Dr. Edward Bach
Wellsprings
Sotwell,
Wallingford,
Berks.

Dear Sir,

We write to acknowledge receipt of your letter
of August 31st and to thank you for £5 cheque enclosed,
towards expense of the printing and distribution of
leaflets.

"THE TWELVE HEALERS" press proofs were passed a week
ago but we 'phoned our printers urgently to postpone the
machining because we were negotiating for the taking of
other premises which provide us with shop accomodation
in a still more central position. We may be in a position
to sign the lease this week and it is preferable,
therefore, to wait and have the new imprint on the new
edition of your booklet. Printing will not be delayed
beyond the beginning of next week and publication will
take place on September 14th.

Yours sincerely

Cumming

Sept.3.1936.

Messrs Daniel.
Ref. CWD/M.

Dear Sirs,

Re Third Edition "The Twelve Healers".

Many thanks for your letter received this morning, and I note with pleasure and satisfaction the date of publication (Sept. 24th.)

Will you please send me as early as possible, three dozen copies with Invoice.

May we wish you every success and a very happy future in your new Headquarters should you make the change.

Yours sincerely.

EDWARD BACH

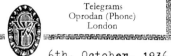

THE C. W. DANIEL COMPANY Ltd.

DIRECTORS: C. W. DANIEL   D. M. WALTHAM

46 Bernard Street, London, W.C.1

(Opposite Russell Square Tube Station)

Telephone
Terminus
4691

Telegrams
Oprodan (Phone)
London

6th. October, 1936.

Ref: CWD/G
Dr. Edward Bach,
Wellsprings,
Sotwell,
Wallingford,
Berkshire.

Dear Dr. Bach,

    We are pleased to hear that you are now
entering upon your lecture campaign and we
hope that it will be successful, and fruitful
of sales of "THE TWELVE HEALERS".

    We should like to be given the sight
of the lecture and the opportunity to submit it
to the Editorial Board of "HEALTH AND LIFE"
with a view to its publication.

Yours sincerely,

C W Daniel

October 22.1936.

Dear Mr. Daniel,

I cannot tell you how pleased I am that your firm is sufficiently interested in our work to wish to publish some account of it.

The healing being effected with these Herbs is nothing short of miraculous, and the fame of them is spreading all over the world.

I am confident that any journal which undertook to publish information concerning these Remedies, and would accept articles written by those who had seen their power to relieve suffering, that journal could not fail. It would be a subject which would supply an ever-increasing publicity.

As the one who was privileged to be shown these Remedies, I can say little more. There are others who would bear testimony. But during now nearly ten years, the success which has attended their use, has surpassed the hopes and expectations of even those who have devoted their lives in this cause, to relieve the sick.

Yours very gratefully for all you and your firm have done for us.

EDWARD BACH

Part Two

Following the publication of his final work, Dr. Bach immediately turned his attention to the broadcast of his findings by way of a lecture tour. The first of these took place on his fiftieth birthday, 24th September 1936 at the Masonic Hall in Wallingford.

Public Lecture

IN THE

MASONIC HALL, WALLINGFORD,

ON

Thursday, Sept. 24th

AT 8 P.M.,

1936

Healing by Herbs

For use in every Home,

BY

Dr. EDWARD BACH.

ADMISSION FREE.

S. BRADFORD, PRINTER, ST. MARY'S STREET, WALLINGFORD.

INTRODUCTION.

From the earliest times in history, we find that herbs have been used as healing remedies, and as far back as records go, man has had the faith that in the herbs of the meadow and valley and hillside lay the power to cure his illnesses. Hundreds of years before Christ, the ancient Indians and Arabians and other races were experts in the use of Nature's gifts; also the early Egyptians, and later the Greeks and Romans, and in a lesser degree right on up till our time.

Now, it is not likely that for thousands of years, great nations of different creeds and colours should have continuously believed in, and persistently studied and used the Herbs of Nature as cures, unless behind it all there was a great truth.

In olden days, not only the physicians of the countries used and taught the use of herbs, but the people themselves had great knowledge of their virtue, and were able to care for themselves in many cases of disorders.

This country is no exception, although at the present time the use of natural means is not so general; yet, until but a generation or two ago, and even today in the more remote parts of the land, households possess their own herbal chest and cures for their household illnesses.

There have been different books written in England during the last four or five hundred years on Herbal Healing; one of the last and most famous is Kulpepper's, written some three hundred years ago.

This book you can still find, studied and used and highly prized in the more country homes of the British Isles, and though it contains the account of over 300 herbs, which must mean much study, yet such is the faith still living that people take the trouble to master it and treat most of their own complaints.

During history there have been times, when disease was successfully dealt with by practically herbs alone; at other times the great and natural art of healing has largely been forgotten: this is one of those times. But such is the power of Nature's way, that it is certain to return to us.

In olden times when a great nation disappeared, much of its learning was lost with it; but now, since discoveries are made at once much more universal, there is hope that the blessings bestowed upon us, as they are rediscovered, will be spread worldwide and so always safely preserved in some country. The herbs spoken of in this lecture, although but recently discovered, are already being used widely in very many parts of the world.

It is certain that at those times when the right herbs were known and used, wonderful healing results must have been general, and the people of those ages must have had very great faith in them: unless this were so, the fame, the faith, the belief of cure placed in herbs, would not have survived the rise and fall of empires, and been continuously in the minds of people for hundreds and thousands of years.

Healing with the clean, pure, beautiful agents of Nature is surely the one method of all which appeals to most of us, and deep down in our inner self, surely there is something about it that rings true indeed: something which tells us – this is Nature's way and is right.

To Nature we look confidently for all the needs to keep us alive – air, light, food, drink, and so on: it is not likely that in this great scheme which provides all, the healing of our illnesses and distress should be forgotten.

So we see that Herbal treatment goes back to the very earliest times known to man; that it has continued all these centuries both in use and in fame, and at many times in history has been the chief and almost the only method of healing.

The system being spoken of this evening has great advantages over others.

Firstly. All the remedies are made from beautiful flowers, plants and trees of Nature: none of them are poisonous nor can do any harm, no matter how much was taken.

Secondly. They are only 38 in number, which means that it is easier to find the right herb to give, than when there are very many.

Thirdly. The method of choosing which remedies to give is simple enough for most people to understand.

Fourthly. The cures which have been obtained have been so wonderful, that they have passed all expectations of even those who use this method, as well as the patients who have received the benefit.

These herbs have succeeded again and again where all other treatment, which has been tried, has failed.

And now, having given you some idea of how ancient and renowned is the great art of healing the suffering by means of herbs, let us pass on to the main reason of this evening's address.

PART 2.

The main objects of this evening's lecture are two:

Firstly: to describe to you a new method of herbal healing.

Secondly: to reduce as much as possible any fear that any of you may have of disease.

Although it is but some seven years ago since the first of a series of the 38 herbs, which are the subject of this address, was discovered, yet in that short time these herbs have been proved to have the most wonderful power of healing. This proof has been found not only in this country, not only in countries on the Continent, but in lands as far distant as India, America, New Zealand, Australia and so on.

It is impossible to tell you of the very great number of people who have had benefit and cures, because they are scattered almost world-wide: but this we know, that hundreds and thousands of sufferers have received help which they had not thought was possible, and beyond any hope which had been left in them.

The important points of treatment with these herbs are:

1. that the remedies are all made from beautiful plants and trees of Nature, and that none of them are hurtful nor can they do any harm.

2. that without a knowledge of medicine their use can be understood so easily that they can be used in the household. Think a moment what this means. There are amongst us in almost every town or village some who have to a lesser or greater degree the desire to be able to help in illness; to be able to relieve the suffering and heal the sick, but from circumstances have been prevented from becoming doctors or nurses, and have not felt that they were able to carry out their desire or mission.

These herbs place in their hands the power to heal amongst their own families, friends and all around them.

In addition to their occupation, they are enabled in their spare time to do a very great amount of good, as many are so doing today; and there are some who have even given up their work to devote all their time to this form of healing.

It means to those who always had an ideal, a dream of relieving the suffering, that it has been made possible for them, whether it be but their own household or on a wider scale.

Again to impress upon you that there is no need of scientific knowledge necessary when treating with these herbs: not even the name of the illness or disease is required. It is not the disease that matters: it is the patient. It is not what the patient has. It is not the disease, so-called, that really is the important thing to treat; because the same disease may cause different results in different people. If the effects were always the same in all people, it would be easy to know what the name of the disease was: but this is not so; and this is the reason why often in medical science it is so difficult to give a name to the particular complaint from which a patient is suffering.

It is not the disease that is of importance. It is the patient; the way in which he or she is affected which is our true guide to healing.

In ordinary every day life, everyone of us has a character of our own.

This is made up of our likes, our dislikes, our ideas, thoughts, wishes, ambitions, the way we treat others, and so on.

Now this character is not of the body, it is of the mind; and the mind is the most delicate and sensitive part of ourselves. So can we wonder that the mind with its various moods will be the first to show the symptoms of disease; and being so sensitive, will be a much better guide to us in illness than depending on the body.

Changes in our minds will guide us clearly to the remedy we need; when the body may show little alteration.

Now let us turn our attention to some of the different ways in which one particular complaint can affect an individual.

We all know the same illness may take us quite differently: if Tommy gets measles, he may be irritable – Sissy may be quiet and drowsy – Johnny wants to be petted – little Peter may be all nerves and fearful – Bobbie wants to be left alone, and so on.

Now, if the disease has such different effects, it is certain it is no use treating the disease alone; it is better to treat Tommy, Sissy, and Johnny and Peter and Bobbie and get them each well, and 'goodbye' the measles.

What it is important to impress upon you, is that it is not the measles which gives the guide to the cure, but it is the way the little one is affected: and the mood of the little one is the most sensitive guide as to know what that particular patient needs.

And just as moods guide us to the treatment in illness, so also they may warn us ahead of a complaint approaching and enable us to stop the attack.

Little Tommy comes home from school unusually tired, or drowsy, or irritable, or wanting to be fussed, or perhaps left alone and so on. He is 'not quite himself' as we say. Kind neighbours come in and say, 'Tommy is sickening for something, you will have to wait'. But why wait: if Tommy is treated then according to his mood, he may very soon again be turned from 'not quite himself' into 'quite himself', when whatever illness was threatened will not occur.

And so with any of us: before almost all complaints there is usually a time of not being quite fit or a bit run down: that is the time to treat our condition, get fit and stop things going further.

Prevention is better than cure, and these remedies help us in a wonderful way to get well, and to protect ourselves from attack of things unpleasant.

So much for the earliest stages of disease. Now let us think about those who have been ill for some time, or even a long time. There is again every reason to be hopeful of benefit, either improvement or recovery. Never let anyone give up hope of getting well: such wonderful improvements and such marvellous recoveries have happened with the use of these herbs, even in those in which it was considered hopeless that anything could be done; that to despair is no longer necessary.

Chronic invalids have been restored to a life of usefulness, attended with a return of much happiness and a better and brighter outlook on life in general.

Do not let anyone be frightened at the name given to any disease; after all, what is in a name: and there is no disease of itself which is incurable. This can be asserted, because those suffering from those types of complaints whose names are most dreaded and feared have become well. If some patients have done this, so can others. It takes less time occasionally to cure a so-called terrible illness in some, than one considered less severe in others. It depends more on the individual than the illness.

Now, it is just the same principle of treatment in long illness as when it is slight and short or only even threatened.

Because in a complaint which has been going on for some time we still have our characters; our wishes, hopes, ideas, likes, dislikes and so on.

So again all that is required is to take notice how a patient is being affected by the illness; if there is depression, hopelessness of getting well, fear of becoming worse, irritability, wanting companionship, desire to be quiet and alone, and so on; and to choose the remedy or remedies suitable for the different moods.

And it is wonderful here again, that just as in threatened illness, if we can get a patient back from being 'not quite themselves', the disease will not happen; so in cases which have been going on for a long time, as the various moods, depression, fear etc, disappear, so the patients are better in themselves, more like their real selves, and with this the disease, no matter what it may be, goes also.

There is yet another class of people, quite different: those who are not really ill in the ordinary sense of the word; yet are always having something wrong with them; perhaps not serious, yet quite enough to make life a trial and a burden at times, and who would be grateful indeed to be rid of their complaints. Mostly they have tried many things to be free of their trouble, but have not been able to find a cure.

Amongst such are those who have frequent headaches; others are subject to severe colds each year; some suffer from catarrh, or rheumatics, or indigestion, or eye-strain, or asthma, or slight heart-trouble, sleeplessness, and so on, whatever it may be.

And what a joy it is to be able to give such people relief: when often they had expected they would have to bear their infirmity all their life; and especially to those who had dreaded that their symptoms might get worse with age. Such cases can be cured and very often benefit begins soon after treatment has started.

And lastly, one more class: people who are quite well, strong and healthy, and yet have their difficulties.

Such people who find their work or play made more difficult from things like: over-anxiety to do right, or too enthusiastic, and strain and tire themselves: or those who fear failure, imagining themselves not as clever as other people: or those unable to make up their minds as to what they want: those who are afraid something will happen to those dear to them, who always fear the worst, even without any reason: those who are too active and restless and never seem at peace: those who are too sensitive and shy and nervous, and so on. All such things, though they may not be called illnesses, cause unhappiness and worry: yet all these can be put right and an added joy comes into life.

So we see how great is the power of the right herbs to heal; not only to keep us strong and protect us from disease, not only to stop an illness when it is threatened, not only to relieve and cure us when we may be in distress and ill, but even to bring peace and happiness and joy to our minds when there is apparently nothing wrong with our health.

Once again, let it be made quite certain that, whether it is being run down, or not quite oneself; whether trying to prevent a disease; whether it is a short illness or a long, the principle is the same – treat the patient; treat the patient according to the mood, according to the character, the individuality, and you can not go wrong.

Think once again the joy this brings, to any one who wants to be able to do something for those who are ill, to be able to help even those where medical science can do no more; it gives to them the power to be healers amongst their fellows.

Yet again, think what a different outlook this brings into our lives; the loss of fear, and the increase of hope.

This work of healing has been done, and published and given freely so that people like yourselves can help yourselves, either in illness or to keep well and strong. It requires no science; only a little knowledge and sympathy and understanding of human nature, which is usual with almost all of us.

THE REMEDIES.

There is not time this evening to give you an outline of the whole 38 Remedies. And it is not entirely necessary, because if you understand the way in which three or four are used you have the principle which applies to them all.

So we will consider the Remedies which are given in case of FEAR.

It does not matter whether it is an accident, sudden illness, a long illness or even in those who are quite well in themselves. If fear is present, one of the Remedies for fear should be given.

Of course, other Remedies may be required at the same time, as there may be other conditions present, then they would be given in addition; but that depends on the case.

Fear is very common in some form or other: not only amongst the ill, but amongst ourselves who otherwise may be well. But whatever it may be, the

Remedies will help us to be free of that great burden which we call fear.

There are five types of fear, and therefore there are five Remedies, one for each type.

The first is when the fear is very great, amounting to terror or panic: either in the patient or because the condition is so serious as to cause intense fear to those around. It may be in case of sudden illness, or accident, but always when there is great emergency or danger, give the Remedy for this: made from a small plant which is called ROCK ROSE.

It is a beautiful thing with a bright yellow flower, it grows on hillsides often where the ground is stony or rocky; and a cultivated variety is to be found on rockeries in gardens, though the one growing naturally should always be chosen for healing.

This Remedy has had wonderful results, and many an alarming case has been better within minutes or hours of its being given.

The key-notes for this Remedy are:

Panic, terror, great emergency or danger.

The second kind of fear is more common: and is the one which applies to everyday life.

The ordinary fears so many of us get. Fear of accidents, fear of illness, fear of a complaint getting worse, fear of the dark, of being alone, of burglars, or fire, of poverty, of animals, of other people and so on. Fears of definite things, whether there be any reason or not.

The Remedy for this is a beautiful plant called MIMULUS: rather like Musk. Some summers it grows in the stream at Ewelme, which runs alongside the road.

The third kind of fear is of those vague unaccountable things which cannot be explained. As if something dreadful is going to happen, without any idea as to what it may be.

All such dreads for which no reason can be

given, and yet are very real and disturbing to the individual, require the Remedy of the ASPEN TREE. And the relief which this has brought to many is truly wonderful.

The fourth kind of fear is that when there is a dread of the mind being over-worked, and the fear that it cannot stand the strain.

When impulses come upon us to do things we should not in the ordinary way think about or for one moment consider.

The Remedy for this comes from the CHERRY PLUM, which grows in the hedge-rows around this district. This drives away all the wrong ideas and gives the sufferer mental strength and confidence.

Lastly, the fifth kind is the fear for others, especially those dear to us.

If they return late, there is the thought that some accident must have happened: if they go for a holiday, the dread that some calamity will befall them. Some illnesses become very serious complaints, and there is great anxiety even for those who are not dangerously ill. Always fearing the worst and always anticipating misfortune for them.

The Remedy made from the RED CHEST-NUT BLOSSOM, of the tree so well known to all of us, soon removes such fears and helps us to think more normally.

It is not easy to confuse these five different kinds of fear, as they are quite distinct; and although fear is the commonest mood we have to treat, it requires but one or more of five Remedies to combat it in all its forms.

Amongst the other Remedies, you will find those which apply to all the conditions that can be met. Such as some for those who suffer from uncertainty, never knowing quite what they wish or what is right for them. Some for loneliness. Others for those who are too sensitive. Others for depression, and so on.

And with very little effort it becomes easy to

find the Remedy or Remedies which a patient needs to help them.

And, once again, the important point is this: that wonderful as it may seem, relieve your patient of the mood or moods such as are given in this system of healing, and your patient is better.

Masonic Lecture

1936.

INTRODUCTION.

I am not going to attempt this evening to give you any details of the wonderful Herbs which are the subject of this address. All that you can obtain from the book.

The main principles are these:

Firstly.   That no medical knowledge whatever is required.

Secondly.   That the disease itself is of no consequence whatsoever.

Thirdly.   That the mind is the most sensitive part of our bodies, and hence the best guide to tell us what remedy is required.

Fourthly.   Thus the manner in which a patient reacts to an illness is alone taken into account. Not the illness itself.

Fifthly.   That such as: fear, depression, doubt, hopelessness, irritability, desire for company or desire to be alone, indecision, such are the true guides to the way in which a patient is being affected by his malady, and to the Remedy which he needs.

There is no need to tell you of the Great Healing Properties of these Remedies, more than to say that hundreds and thousands of people have been brought back to health who had no hope of anything but life-long malady. And vast numbers have been quickly cured of ordinary illness: and again, vast numbers have had disease prevented in its early stages.

Moreover the fame of these Herbs is such that they are not only being used in these Islands, but in most of the countries of the world.

The whole principle of Healing by this

method is so simple as can be understood by almost everyone, and even the very Herbs themselves can be gathered and prepared by any who take delight in such.

PART 2.

Brethren, we are taught that within us dwells a Vital and Immortal Principle.

Man throughout all the centuries of which we have history has believed that there was something within himself, greater and more wonderful than his body, and which lived on after the grave.

This belief has been in the mind of man from time immemorial.

We are all conscious that it is not our bodies alone which are the cause of our difficulties. We do not say, "my body is worried or anxious or depressed"; we say, "I am worried or anxious or depressed". We do not say, "my hand hurts itself in pain"; we say, "my hand hurts me".

Were we but bodies, our lives would be merely one of personal interest and gain, seeking but our own comforts and relieving our own needs.

But this is not so. Every kindly smile, every kindly thought and action; every deed done for love or sympathy or compassion of others proves that there is something greater within us than that we see. That we carry a Spark of the Divine, that within us resides a Vital and Immortal principle.

And the more that Spark of Divinity shines within us, the more our lives radiate Its sympathy, Its compassion and Its love, the more we are beloved by our fellow-men and fingers are pointed at us and the words are said, "There goes a God-like man".

Moreover, the amount of peace, of happiness, of joy, of health and of well-being that comes into our lives depends also on the amount of which the Divine Spark can enter and illuminate our existence.

From time immemorial, man has looked at two great sources for Healing. To his Maker, and to the Herbs of the field, which his Maker has placed for the relief of those who suffer.

Yet one Truth has mostly been forgotten. That those Herbs of the field placed for Healing, by comforting, by soothing, by relieving our cares, our anxieties, bring us nearer to the Divinity within. And it is that increase of the Divinity within which heals us.

It is a very wonderful thought, but it is absolutely true, that certain Herbs, by bringing us solace, bring us closer to our Divinity: and this is shewn again and again in that the sick not only recover from their malady, but in so doing, peace, hope, joy, sympathy and compassion enter into their lives; or if these qualities had been there before, become much increased.

Thus we can truly say that certain Herbs have been placed for us by Divine Means, and the help which they give to us, not only heals our bodies, but brings into our lives, our characters, attributes of our Divinity.

So in healing with these Herbs, the body is not taken into any account; whatever may be wrong with it is of no consideration. All we seek are those characters of the sufferer where he is in disharmony with the Well of Peace in his Soul.

Thus the ordinary symptoms of the flesh are ignored, and all thought is given to such things as depression, impatience, worry, fear, indecision, anxiety, doubt, intolerance, condemnation and so on. All those qualities which are absent in the stillness, the certainty, the compassion of our Inner Selves.

And as by treatment with the Divine Herbs of Healing these adverse qualities will disappear, so with their disappearance, no matter what the disease, the body becomes well.

It is as though in this vast civilisation of today, a civilisation of great stress and strain, the turmoil has been such that we have become too far parted from the true Source of Healing, Our Divinity. Yet our Maker, knowing these things, took compassion upon us, and in His Mercy provided a substitute means to heal our infirmities until when time or circumstance shall restore the genuine and direct.

Yet these substituted means are wonderful in their help: for to see the joy, the happiness, the tenderness that comes into life after life as the Herbs heal them, prove beyond doubt that, not the body alone has received blessing.

Moreover, it is certain that it is increased harmony between the Greater Self within and the body without which has affected the cure.

There is no need to go into detail of the whole 38: that can be obtained from the book. Suffice it to say that there is one for every mood which can be an opposition to our happy joyful selves. And all that is necessary is to know that mood or moods present in the patient and give the Remedy or Remedies which remove them.

It does not matter whether the illness is of only a few minutes or of many years duration, the principle is the same.

Moreover, consider what this means in everyday life. Nearly all of us have some trait which is out of harmony, such as depression, worry, fear and so on. These Herbs remove such and by so doing not only close the door to the entrance of disease, but make our lives happier, more joyous and more useful.

And what greater is there amongst all the Noble Arts than that of Healing. And what more befitting to the Brotherhood of Man than, like some of the Orders of Old, to carry ease to those in pain; solace to those in trial or distress; and comfort and hope to all those afflicted.

And these Remedies place in the hands of

everyone the power to do these things. Not of their own power, but of the Power vested by the Great Creator in His Healing Herbs.

Part Three

The following collection of letters completes this final chapter in Dr. Bach's life. They were written during his last month, and because he knew that it would not be long before he was to leave his earthly existence behind, his letters speak of how and by whom his work should continue.

He wrote to Mr. Daniel, his publisher, whom he had never met, requesting that any profits from the sale of the books, which would continue to fund the work, should be sent to Nora Weeks, explaining that she, as his fellow-worker, was expertly conversant with all aspects of the work and would therefore be responsible for its future.

Dr. Bach knew Nora well and was certain that she had the necessary qualities to wholeheartedly protect the purity of the work, and so it was into her safe hands, with the help of the other team members, that Dr. Bach firmly placed the continuity and care of the work he founded.

> *"His work of healing with these Herbs is being continued, at his expressed wish, by his own Team of workers at the headquarters of the work at Sotwell, and his own principle of charging no fees to any patient is being continued also."*
>
> *Nora Weeks.*

Sadly, over the years, just as Dr. Bach predicted, there have been numerous attempts to change his original work – to extend it, "bring it up to date", or "improve" his methods of prescribing. Even Dr. Bach himself was subjected to such persuasive attempts and it is about one such matter that he wrote to Victor Bullen. (On that occasion, there was a persistent suggestion that all 38 remedies should be combined together, despite the fact that Dr. Bach had disproved this idea.) In that letter, he emphasised the importance of upholding the simplicity of the work, and that although attempts to distort or destroy it would be made, it was their work to steadfastly adhere to its purity.

Since Nora and Victor's passing, it has now become OUR work to uphold these principles, and we too must be steadfast in our endeavours to ensure that Dr. Bach's work remains intact and as straightforward as he intended.

October 26.1936.

Dear Folk,
      It would be wonderful to form a little Brotherhood without rank or office, none greater and none less than the other, who devoted themselves to the following principles:

      1. That there has been disclosed unto us a system of Healing such as has not been known within the memory of man; when, with the simplicity of the Herbal remedies, we can set forth with the certainty, the ABSOLUTE CERTAINTY, of their power to conquer disease.

      2. That we never criticise nor condemn the thoughts, the opinions, the ideas of others; ever remembering that all Humanity are God's children, each striving in his own way to find the Glory of The Father.

      3. That we set out on the one hand, as Knights of old, to destroy the dragon of fear, knowing that we may never have one discouraging word, but that we can bring HOPE aye, and most of all, CERTAINTY to those who suffer.

      4. That we never get carried away by praise or success that we meet in our mission, knowing that we are but the messengers of the Great Power.

      5. That as more and more we gain the confidence of those around, we proclaim to them we believe that we are Divine agents sent to succour them in their need.

6. That as people become well, that the Herbs of the field, which are healing them, are the gift of Nature which is the Gift of God; thus bringing them back to a belief in the LOVE, the MERCY, the tender COMPASSION and the ALMIGHTY POWER of THE MOST HIGH.

EDWARD BACH

Mount Vernon,
Sotwell, Wallingford,
Berks.

October 26.1936.

Dear Vic,

I think now you have seen every phase of the Work.

This last episode of Doctor Max Wolf may be welcomed. It is a proof of the value of our Work when material agencies arise to distort it, because the distortion is a far greater weapon than attempted destruction.

As soon as a teacher has given his work to the world, a contorted version of the same must arise.

Such has happened even from the humblest like ourselves, who have dedicated our services to the good of our fellow-men, even to the Highest of all, the Divinity of Christ.

The contortion must be raised for people to be able to choose between the gold and the dross.

Our work is steadfastly to adhere to the simplicity and purity of this method of healing; and when the next edition of The Twelve Healers becomes necessary, we must have a longer introduction, firmly upholding the harmlessness, the simplicity, and the miraculous healing powers of the Remedies, which have been shown to us through a greater Source than our own intellects.

I feel now, dear brother, that as I find it more and more necessary to go into temporary solitude, you have the whole situation in hand and can cope with all matters either connected with patients or connected with the administration of this work of healing, knowing that people like ourselves who have tasted the glory of self-sacrifice, the glory of helping our brothers, once we have been given a jewel of such magnitude, nothing can deviate us from our path of love and duty to displaying its lustre, pure and unadorned to the people of the world.

Sotwell,
Wallingford, BERKS.

November 1.1936.

Dear Mr Daniel,

I am daily expecting a call to a work more congenial than of this very difficult world.

The point is, should there be any profits from the sale of the books credited to my name, would you send them to Miss Nora Grey Weeks, of, for the moment, the above address. She has been my fellow-worker for many years, and can advise you in any case of difficulty about this work.

She has helped me collect the Herbs, she has studied with me their possibilities, and knows all I know about the work.

Dear Mr Daniel, when we are on the verge of passing through the Valley of the Shadow, perhaps we are not so reserved as we are at a rummage sale, especially when we have had a brandy or two to buck us up.

The Work I have put before you is Great Work, is God's Work, and heaven only knows why I should be called away at this moment to continue to fight for suffering humanity.

EDWARD BACH

November 1.1936.

Dear Lovely People,

There are moments such as this when I am expecting a summons to where I know not.

But if that call comes as it may any minute, I do plead with you, you three, to carry on the wonderful Work we have started. A Work that can rob disease of its power, the Work which can set men free.

What I have attempted to write, should be added to the introduction of the next edition of "The Twelve Healers".

EDWARD BACH

August 21.1939.

Dear Mr Daniel,

Enclosed the alterations and additions which Dr. Bach himself suggested in the next edition of "The Twelve Healers and Other Remedies."

The new part of the introduction he wished to be inserted at the beginning, and the present introduction to follow on immediately.

I hope this is all quite clear, but we can always correct it in the proof you send us.

Yours sincerely,

NORA WEEKS

Dictated by Doctor Edward Bach. October 30th 1936.

To be inserted in the next edition of

"THE TWELVE HEALERS"
"AND OTHER REMEDIES"

at the beginning of the present introduction.

INTRODUCTION.

———————————

This system of treatment is the most perfect which has been given to mankind within living memory.

It has the power to cure all disease; and, in its simplicity, it may be used in the household.

It is its simplicity, combined with its all-healing effects, that is so wonderful.

No science, no knowledge is necessary, apart from the simple methods described herein.

And they who will obtain the greatest benefit from this God-sent Gift will be those who keep it pure as it is; free from science, free from theories; for everything in Nature is simple.

This system of healing, which has been Divinely revealed unto us, shows that it is our fears, our cares, our anxieties and such like that open the path to the invasion of illness.

And so by treating our fears, our cares, our worries and so on, we not only free ourselves from our illness, but the Herbs given unto us by the Grace of the Creator of all, in addition take away our fears and worries, and leave us happier and better in ourselves.

As the Herbs heal our fears, our anxieties, our worries, our faults and our failings, it is these we must seek, and then the disease, no matter what it may be, will leave us.

There is little more to say, for the understanding mind will know all this, and may there be sufficient of those with understanding minds, unhampered by the trend of science, to use these Gifts of God for the relief and the blessing of those around them.

And thus, behind all disease lie our fears, our anxieties, our greed, our likes and our dislikes. Let us seek these out and heal them, and with the healing of them will go the disease of which we suffer.

CHAPTER V

REFLECTIONS OF EDWARD BACH

In this chapter we have brought together a selection of character portraits by Dr. Bach's colleagues and friends, together with some photographs taken in his younger days. Dr. Bach loved poetry, Rudyard Kipling in particular, so we have also included a selection of his favourite poems, and we are sure you will enjoy them too.

The character portraits, especially that by Nora Weeks, provide a picture of Dr. Bach's deeper nature and help us to appreciate that he was as human as the rest of us, despite his special purpose in life. He was the most humble man, and knew that he was only a channel through which the healing flowers of Nature could be found. He did not want to be idolised or revered – he felt it was the work that was of importance, not he – he was concerned only with the health and happiness of his fellow brothers and sisters.

Nonetheless, we have so much to be thankful to him for, and to his team of helpers who dedicated their lives to his work. It is indeed a great privilege to be so closely involved with Dr. Bach's work, and a delight to have known and worked with his closest friends and colleagues, Nora Weeks and Victor Bullen. They were indeed very fortunate to have known Dr. Bach personally, and we are most grateful to them, and to all his other dear friends, who have shared their experiences so that we too might know him a little better.

Edward Bach by Nora Weeks.

During the years after Dr. Bach left London to develop this method of healing with the flower Remedies, his sensitivity and inner knowledge became greater and greater, indeed towards the last two years of his life, he was conscious that his hold on the physical body was very tenuous. he had been a vegetarian for many years, but then he felt he must 'coarsen' himself in order to stay in the body until his work was finished. So he ate meat.

He smoked cigarettes quite heavily except when he was listening to that 'inner small voice'. Then there was a radiance about him, as though a light shone around him and the expression of peace on his face was beautiful. This radiance and peace enveloped all who were with him at that time.

He could on occasion too 'turn on' a great enveloping Love. Not a personal love but what seemed to those around the great impersonal Love of the Creator. It had a healing indescribable effect on those around, an enveloping security, joyousness and peace not of this world. He could 'shut it off' in an instant.

And as the personalities of the great souls who come to earth in a body to do special work are of no account – it is their mission which is all important – at times Edward Bach could be angry, irritable, almost brutal in his manner. This did not last long, and with all great souls, he would suffer physically, sometimes agonizingly, from the slightest deviation from the path of compassion and love he had come to travel. Great poets, musicians, artists, Masters, Winston Churchill, had no time to waste on correcting the defects of their personalities, their mission in life occupied all their energies.

Edward Bach 'knew' how people were feeling, no matter how they tried to hide their feelings, and with those who lived with him, at times it made life dificult for them and for him. He would give one look at them and then walk out of the house for the day. He used to say "If you think I am a fool, say so, don't just think it, that hurts too much'. We forget how our inner feelings radiate hurtful radiations.

There were certain people and certain diseases (unless the sufferer had come for help) from whom he had to run away. During the years he was studying human types and states of mind, he would go into restaurants, theatres, cinemas, shops and amongst crowds. often he would have to leave hurriedly as someone there, as he said, was too dominant, too full of hatred or resentment and these negative radiations hit him like a cannonball. Once on

Brighton pier listening to a concert, he got up suddenly with a shout and pelted down the pier. When asked what was the reason, he said "What was that evil thing behind me?" the Man sitting behind him was too all appearances a normal man, but he sensed and reacted to that man's inner feelings.

Often he would be in a state of collapse after seeing certain people, grey in the face, reeling like a drunken man or had to lie down on the grass verge to recover. We often went to look for him and bring him home to recover.

He said he would not protect himself from these experiences, although he could have done so, for he must keep his sensitivity to finish his work as his time was short. He would then have a period of rest and peace, just as Jesus would go away from the crowds for a time for refreshment and strength.

At times he would pass into some wonderful realm and appear to be asleep. He had great difficulty in returning and was often reluctant to do so.

He said once to me "are you ever unconscious of your body?" and when I said 'yes', he replied "You do not know how fortunate you are. All my life my body has suffered in some way from pain and discomfort and distress."

But his tortured body did not interfere at any time with his work. One has seen him tramp for miles with ulcerated legs, blinding headaches, agonizing pain from Tic dolevreux. "I must know what pain is like and experience every kind to have a true understanding of what others suffer."

All this sounds as though he were a saint, the ordinary conception of a saint. He was not like that, he had, as mentioned before, a temper and never hesitated to control it, and he did things at times on purpose to shock people, and he treated those who came out of curiosity, very arbiterally and often with rudeness from the ordinary conventional point of view. Many did not understand him.

On the other hand he had a great sense of humour and enjoyed the simple things of life, which are the true things of life. Picking the first wild mushrooms of the year made him as excited as a boy. Cooking a meal, making a pair of trousers, finishing a chair or table he had made, filled him with joy.

Not only had he an affinity with the plants and trees and bushes, but also with animals. Birds would come to him and perch on the spade with which he was digging and bring their babies with them, fierce dogs would come and lick his hands. If he held a flower in his hand, not only would he know its helpful properties, but he would learn its history. The sea convululous for instance, mauve in colour, told him it grew by the sea to be cleansed and regain its pure white colour, for once it had grown where much blood had been shed, and its petals had been stained with red.

He did remember, although it meant little to him, certain details of his past incarnations. He had always been a healer. Once he saw a picture of himself preparing bottles of healing herbs. So precious were these bottles that they were placed on a shelf and must be so little touched by hand that the labels with the names of the herbs were stuck to the shelves below.

Another time he saw himself plunging into a river to cleanse himself completely, physically and mentally, from his last patient before seeing the next one.

He followed his intuition, 'The inner' urge at all times. What others feel was a trivial thing and not worth while, leaving a good meal on the table, or some interesting conversation, was for him a command. If he felt the urge to go out he would go immediately whatever he was doing. Two occasions come to mind. In the middle of dictating letters in Cromer one time, he left the house and walked towards the pier. On the way he met a man pacing up and down in great distress. Dr. Bach knew him and asked him what was the matter. "I am going to commit suicide, I can't stand it any longer. I am making up my mind to throw myself off the end of the pier." Dr. Bach was able to dissuade him, later to his great gratitude, for his problems were solved quite soon afterwards.

Another day the Doctor suddenly left the luncheon table and walked to the far end of the beach to see a man walking fully clothed into the sea. Another attempt at suicide. Again this man was saved from ending his life.

"Out of the mouths of babes and sucklings." The Doctor listened with full attention to everything anyone told him. "You never know who they are and what truths they have come to tell you."

Many people would say 'I have only to see him in the distance and I am better.'

Clothes and money of course meant nothing to him. His suits were always made a size larger as he could not bear any tightness on his body and hats were not for him, he never wore one.

The conventional idea of a doctor and a consulting room were not his. He welcomed his patients, made them feel they were important, encouraged them to know healing was for them. One woman with a most distressing and repulsive facial sklin complaint was made so happy for he kissed her on both cheeks, within a few days her skin was clear.

He was privileged to be a channel on healing, though his first consideration was to find the healing flowers. These, he said, could be used by others, whereas he could not pass on the gift of healing, that was in Higher hands.

I was once suffering from a severe attack of bronchitis, he passed his hand once over my back. I was immediately well.

Although the mental difficulties, the individual himself, were all important for the prescribing of the flower Remedies, he could without their saying a word, place his hand over the diseased organ, the strained muscle, often with instantaneous healing.

But he could tell with one look at the sufferer, the negative difficulty, the hidden fear, resentment, jealousy or whatever they might be suffering from and name the Remedy for their healing.

And more important still, tell the sufferer what courage, what love and compassion and understanding lay beneath their difficulties. He could see the true nature of each individual, and would tell them what great people they were and that 'God's children are never afraid.'

His voice held a quality that gave confidence, made one feel one was better, nicer, that one was really of consequence and a far lovelier person that one had believed.

Meeting Edward Bach

Writing about Dr. Bach as I knew him is one of those things I am often asked to do, but it is something which is difficult to achieve. I knew him best when I was 12 years old and memories of that time tend to be a little coloured by imagination. Because, however, these memories are needed in making a picture of a very important man, I have tried to put down a few more of the things I can remember.

First and foremost was the fact that my father, also a doctor and an older man than Dr. Bach, had a great respect for his work. From the time he was working with nosodes onwards Dr. Bach's work was often discussed in our house and we children knew that our parents admired him and what he was doing. He made a few visits to our home and we spent one holiday in Cromer when he was there, it is on these brief contacts that I must draw for memories.

One of the things I remember most clearly was his intense dislike of hypocracy, face saving and convention. He wanted everyone to behave and speak as they felt. He was tremendously sensitive to people and personalities, to such an extent that he refused to meet socially, even for a brief conventional greeting, people of whom he disapproved. There was one occasion when he turned and left the room rather than meet a well thought of and fashionable young surgeon who had come to our house especially to be introduced. Yet he was normally kindness itself to everyone. All he demanded was simplicity and straight forwardness. Apart from this one occasion I never remember him being brusque or unkind to anyone. He did, just the same, expect people to take full responsibility for anything they did or said, and even from children he rejected a conventional half truth.

His friendship with my parents must from time to time have caused them more embarrassment than we children suspected. It was during that holiday in Cromer, when I was 12, that I and one of my sisters expressed a desire to smoke cigarettes. We were having a meal in a restaurant at the time and my parents passed the remark off as silly. Not so Dr. Bach. "If they want to smoke, let them smoke," he said. And he handed us cigarettes and lit them for us. My parents were normally conventional people, unlikely to have allowed us to do such a thing in public, but they took it quite calmly, and curiously enough this desire to smoke vanished quite quickly, no doubt because it ceased to be forbidden. None of the three of us smoked much there after and nowadays only one of us smokes at all, and that only very modestly.

To Dr. Bach it was the forbidding, the frustration that was wrong and this came over so strongly, as I remember it, that none of us had any desire to take advantage of the situation or to show off. That we felt well and "right" in his presence was acknowledged among my sisters and myself without really knowing why. But we knew too that when he argued that we should be permitted to do things like smoking he was really giving us the responsibility for what we did and the childish desire to show off or seek forbidden fruit vanished. It was his deep integrity of purpose that produced this reaction and it is this impression of his personality that remains with me to this day.

Frances Thomas

The White Pony – a case history.

Sotwell, 1935.

The farm hand said he was digging the grave for the pony for he was foaming at the mouth, had not eaten for some days and could hardly stand on his feet. They thought he would be dead within an hour or so.

Then the farm-hand said Dr. Bach came along and said to him 'Can you hold his tongue to one side?'·He did so, and the Doctor took a small bottle out of his pocket and poured it down the pony's throat.

He said to the farm-hand, 'You can fill up the grave. Give the pony his usual food and drink' and went away.

The farm hand did as the Doctor said, the pony ate and drank and completely recovered.

The remedies given are unknown, probably Rock Rose or the Rescue Remedy.

Dedication from "Barrack-Room Ballads"
Rudyard Kipling

Beyond the path of the outmost sun through utter darkness hurled –
Farther than ever comet flared or vagrant star-dust swirled –
Live such as fought and sailed and ruled and loved and made our world.

They are purged of pride because they died; they know the worth of their
bays;

They sit at wine with the Maidens Nine and the Gods of the Elder Days –
It is their will to serve or be still as fitteth Our Father's praise.

'Tis theirs to sweep through the ringing deep where Azrael's outposts are,
Or buffet a path through the Pit's red wrath when God goes out to war,
Or hang with the reckless Seraphim on the rein of a red-maned star.

They take their mirth in the joy of the Earth – they dare not grieve for her
pain.

They know of toil and the end of toil; they know God's Law is plain;
So they whistle the Devil to make them sport who know that Sin is vain.

And oft-times cometh our wise Lord God, master of every trade,
And tells them tales of His daily toil, of Edens newly made;
And they rise to their feet as He passes by, gentlemen unafraid.

To these who are cleansed of base Desire, sorrow and Lust and Shame –
Gods for they knew the hearts of men, men for they stooped to Fame –
Borne on the breath that men call Death, my brother's spirit came.

He scarce had need to doff his pride or slough the dross of Earth –
E'en as he trod that day to God so walked he from his birth,
In simpleness and gentleness and honour and clean mirth.

So cup to lip in fellowship they gave him welcome high
And made him place at the banquet board – the Strong Men ranged thereby,
Who had done his work and held his peace and had no fear to die.

Beyond the look of the last lone star, through open darkness hurled,
Further than rebel comet dared or hiving star-swarm swirled,
Sits he with those that praise our God for that they served His word.

The King's Breakfast

The King asked the Queen, and the Queen asked the Dairymaid:
"Could we have some butter for the Royal slice of bread?"
The Queen asked the Dairymaid, the Dairymaid said "Certainly,
I'll go and tell the cow now before she goes to bed."
The Dairymaid she curtsied, and went and told the Alderney:
"Don't forget the butter for the Royal slice of bread."
The Alderney said sleepily: "You'd better tell His Majesty
That many people nowadays like marmalade instead."
The Dairymaid said, "Fancy!" and went to Her Majesty.
She curtsied to the Queen, and she turned a little red:
"Excuse me, Your Majesty, for taking of the liberty,
But marmalade is tasty, if it's very thickly spread."
The Queen said "Oh!" and went to His Majesty:
"Talking of the butter for the Royal slice of bread,
Many people think that marmalade is nicer.
Would you like to try a little marmalade instead?"
The King said, "Bother!" and then he said,
"Oh, deary me!" The King sobbed, "Oh, deary me!" and went back to bed.
"Nobody," he whimpered, "Could call me a fussy man;
I *only* want a little bit of butter for my bread!"
The Queen said, "There, there!" and went to the Dairymaid.
The Dairymaid said "There, there!" and went to the shed.
The cow said, "There, there! I didn't really mean it;
Here's milk for his porringer and butter for his bread."
The Queen took the butter and brought it to His Majesty;
The King said, "Butter, eh?" and bounced out of bed.
"Nobody," he said, as he kissed her tenderly,
"Nobody," he said as he slid down the banisters,
"Nobody, my darling, could call me a fussy man –
BUT
I *do* like a little bit of butter to my bread!"

A . A. Milne,
from "When we were very young".
Published by Methuen Children's Books.

Under the Wiltshire Apple Tree

Some folk as can afford, so I've heard say,
Set up a sort of cross right in the garden way
      to mind 'em of the Lord.
But I, when I do see t'is apple tree and stooping limb, spread wi' moss,
I think of God and how He trod that garden long ago.
He walked, I reckon, to and fro and then sat down upon the groun',
Or some low limb as suited Him, such as you see on many a tree,
And on t'is very one where I at set o' sun do sit and talk wi' He.
And mornins too I rise and come and sit down where the branches be low.
The birds do sing, the bees do hum, the flowers in the border blow,
And all my heart's so glad and clear, like pools when mists do disappear.
Like pools alaughin' in the light when mornin's air tis all swep and bright.
Like pools wot got Heaven in sight so's my heart's cheer.
He never pushed when He be near the garden door nor left a footmark on the
      floor.
I never heard Un stir nor tread an yet His Hand do bless my head.
And when tis time for work to start I take Him with me in my heart.
And when I die, pray God I see at very last t'is apple tree and stooping limb
And think of Him and all He bin to me.

Anna de Bary.

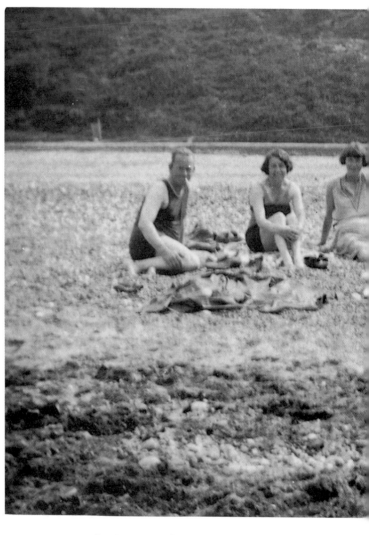

On the beach at Cromer, Norfolk 1932.
Dr. Bach is on the left, Nora Weeks 3rd from left.

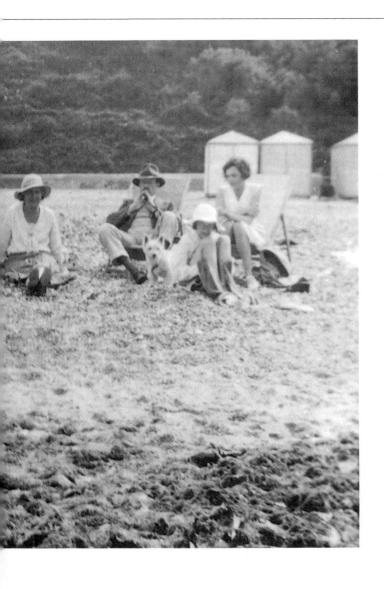

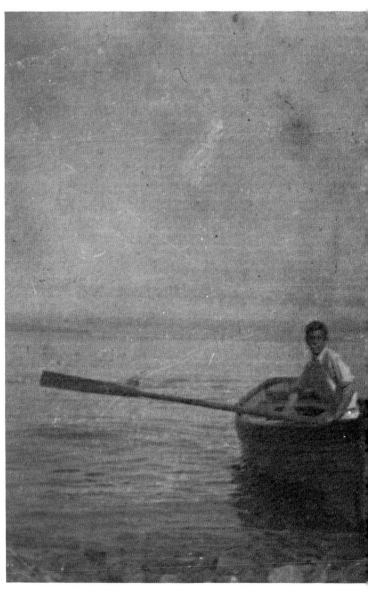

Dr. Bach, aged 19, Wales 1905.

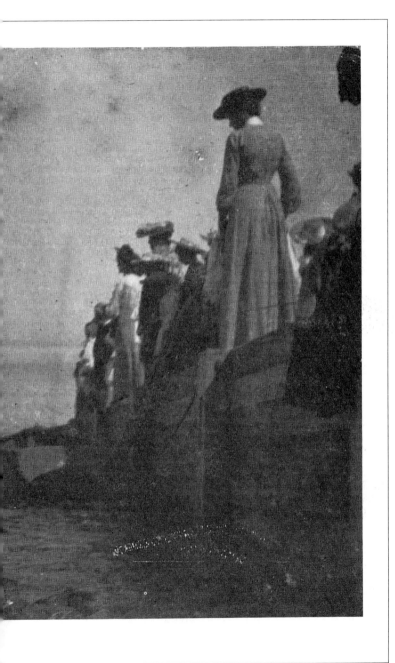

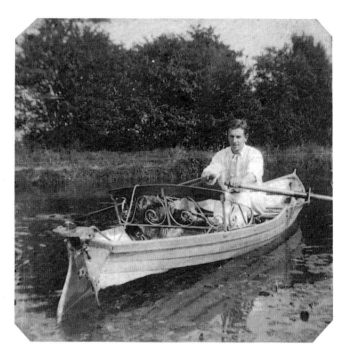

Dr. Bach, aged 19, Wales 1905.

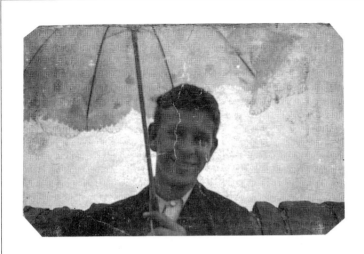

Dr. Bach, aged 19, Wales 1905.

Edward Bach.

Eager and ardent, like a living flame,
Without a thought of self, desiring ever
Nor wealth nor power nor influence nor fame
Except as those might forward his endeavour
To help mankind. So swift to understand
All doubts and fears and failures, yet so slow
To judge or to condemn, he set his hand
Alone to heal, to help those powers to grow
That make for fellowship and cast out hate
And aim to help the whole wide world to gain
Touch with the Infinite. Darkly we wait
So long for light, so oft it seems in vain,
But here was a life that sped too swiftly by
Yet kindled fires that will be slow to die.

C.E.W.

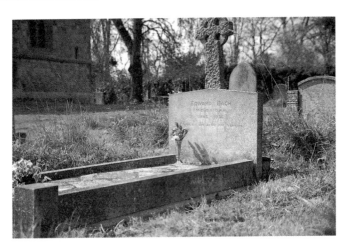

"Behold I am alive for evermore"

Deep Peace of the Running Wave to you,
Deep Peace of the Flowing Air to you,
Deep Peace of the Quiet Earth to you,
Deep Peace of the Shining Stars to you,
Deep Peace of the Son of Peace to you.

Fiona Macleod.

Maria Ryan STAT.
129 Camden Mews
London NW1 9AH.